YOUNG ENDEAVOUR

YOUNG ENDEAVOUR

Contributions to Science by
Medical Students of the Past
Four Centuries

By

WILLIAM CARLETON GIBSON
D.Phil. (Oxon.), M.D., C.M.
Kinsmen Professor of Neurological Research
University of British Columbia

With a Foreword by

SIR HENRY DALE, O.M.

CHARLES C THOMAS • PUBLISHER
Springfield • Illinois • U.S.A.

CHARLES C THOMAS • PUBLISHER
BANNERSTONE HOUSE
301-327 East Lawrence Avenue, Springfield, Illinois, U.S.A.

Published simultaneously in the British Commonwealth of Nations by
BLACKWELL SCIENTIFIC PUBLICATIONS, LTD., OXFORD, ENGLAND

Published simultaneously in Canada by
THE RYERSON PRESS, TORONTO

Library of Congress Catalog Card Number: 58-8419

With THOMAS BOOKS careful attention is given to all details of manufacturing and design. It is the Publisher's desire to present books that are satisfactory as to their physical qualities and artistic possibilities and appropriate for their particular use. THOMAS BOOKS will be true to those laws of quality that assure a good name and good will.

Printed in the United States of America

To the spirit of William Osler
renascent in my teachers

Maude Abbott
W. W. Francis
Wilder Penfield

"History is simply the biography of the mind of man; and our interest in history, and its educational value to us, is directly proportionate to the completeness of our study of the individuals through whom this mind has been manifested."

—William Osler

"(Biography means essentially) the sifting of human creations!—nothing less than this is what we ought to mean by the humanities. . . . *What our colleges should teach is therefore biographical history, that not of politics merely, but of anything and everything so far as human efforts and conquests are factors that have played their parts.* Studying in this way we learn what types of activity have stood the test of time; we acquire standards of the excellent and durable. All our arts and sciences and institutions are but so many quests of perfection on the part of men; and when we see how diverse the types of excellence may be, how various the tests, how flexible the adaptations, we gain a richer sense of what the terms "better" and "worse" may signify in general. Our critical sensibilities grow both more acute and less fanatical. We sympathize with men's mistakes even in the act of penetrating them; and we feel the pathos of lost causes and misguided epochs even while we applaud what overcame them."

William James

Foreword

by

Sir Henry Dale, O.M.

ANYONE who can look back over 60 years or more, to recall his own student days, must surely regard with wonder, as I do daily, the absorptive capacity which any of the rapidly growing branches of natural science must require of its student today; and in no case is this demand more obvious than in that of the scientific disciplines which now contribute to knowledge in the medical range. The course of study required for an effective qualification in medicine is inevitably growing longer; but, if a man is to begin his life's work before he enters the period of natural decline, the duration of his formal studies can certainly not be expected, or even be allowed, to increase in direct proportion to the ever more rapid growth, both in range and volume, of the kinds of knowledge with which he ought still to obtain at least a nodding acquaintance, if he is to be provided with an adequate basis for an intelligent conduct of his practice.

While, however, the demand upon a medical student's time, and upon his innate capacity for learning and retention, is growing thus with an even alarming rapidity, it is evident that opportunities to try his hand at research, and thus to obtain some practical experience of its methods and of the significance of its results, are much more readily available now to the proper kind of interest and enterprise, than they were in the bygone days, when there was so relatively little to be learnt, and when it might, accordingly, have seemed so much easier to spare the time for a diversion from the narrow way of formal education. There were those among us, indeed, who were so fortunate as to receive, even then, some of the rare opportunities which were on offer; and of the medical students of today, there must surely be a larger proportion than ever before, of those who, in spite of the formidable claims of an expanding curriculum, continue still to find time somehow for a practical contact with the methods of research, even though many of them will find little further direct use for that experience, except in connexion with the practical application of medical knowledge. The value, however, of even so brief and tentative a personal experience of the ways of research, must surely continue to increase, in these days when the knowledge applied in medical practice is finding its basis ever more in the results of experimental enquiry, and ever less in the authority of tradition and empiricism, which had continued so largely to dominate it, till times which are well within the memory of some of us who are still living and watching the changing scene today.

This educational value, of an experience of research during the student period, was clearly prominent in Professor Gibson's mind, when he was collecting from a great range of medical history the examples of the important discoveries which have been made by men who were still students of medicine when they made them, and which have provided him with the main substance of this delightfully stimulating book. Towards the end of it he gives us a glimpse of his own uneasy feelings about the threatened effect of the modern curriculum, "over-loading our undergraduates with a phenomenal amount of detail in some subjects. . . ." "Over and above the 'legal minimum' of instruction," he continues, "we face the question of how best to develop the enquiring mind, for this mind surely is the patient's greatest guarantee of good diagnosis and rational treatment." It surely cannot be doubted, that Professor Gibson is rightly concerned about this central problem of medical education today—how to ensure that the student shall continue to acquire a sufficiently competent grasp of what is really essential, out of the mounting superabundance of what is known, and at the same time to sharpen rather than to satiate his appetite for the further developments of knowledge, and to stimulate rather than to quench any spark of imagination, any faculty of mental enterprise, with which nature may have endowed him.

Professor Gibson's own immediate prescription, then, is a wide survey of medical history, in order to bring more clearly to notice, or in some cases, perhaps, to rescue from the threat of oblivion, examples of the kinds of discoveries which have been made by medical students. These discoveries extend, indeed, over a remarkable range of subjects; and they show as wide a range of variety, with respect to the kinds of activity and of claims to distinction and remembrance, which are to be found in the after lives of those who made them while they were still students. We find cases in which these student activities already made clear the natural bent, for what was to become the subject of a life's devotion. Vesalius, we see, began to make in his boyhood, and then continued as a student of medicine, the dissections of all kinds of animals, and the studies of human skeletons, which were to lead directly to his life's great achievement, and to his fame as the first of modern anatomists. And we find here a number of other such examples, of men whose great contributions to the growth of knowledge, whether in medicine, or in other natural sciences, or in an even more generous range, seem to have been continuous with those in which they were already engaged when they were students of medicine, or even earlier. Albrecht von Haller, for example, is said to have made a beginning of his life's work with the "compilation of two thousand biographies from his own pen at 8 years of age." He was clearly, in more than one respect, an infant prodigy; but it is possible that that kind of scholarly instinct, for the industrious and critical assemblage of information, is apt to become evident relatively early in life. Professor Gibson presents us, on the other hand, with many cases of at least equal interest, in which a discovery made at the student stage of a man's career could have offered no definite clue, to the direction of the major contributions which he was to make to knowledge in the course of his main career. Thus Humphry Davy was still a student, in Dr. Beddoes' rather curious "Pneumatic Institution" in Bristol, when he discovered the anaesthetic properties of Nitrous Oxide. This, no doubt, played a part in enabling him to become an assistant, and eventually Professor of Chemistry, in the Royal Institution in London. It was there, we may note in passing, that Davy's own assistant, Michael Faraday, was later to observe the anaesthetic effects of ether, and to recommend it as having advantages for such purposes over nitrous oxide, as early as 1818—some 28 years before its famous first practical application by Morton, in Boston, Massachusetts. It can hardly be suggested, in any case, that Davy's early enterprise in the field of anaesthesia gave any clear hint of the powers which would lead him to such major achievements as the discovery of the metals of the alkalies and alkaline earths. Plenty of other such examples will be found and enjoyed by the readers of this book. Thus, to select only a few more for quotation, we find records of early observations by Edward Jenner on *angina pectoris*, by A. V. Waller on diapedesis in the blood-vessels of the frog's tongue, by Robert Koch on the excretion of succinic acid, by Victor Horsley on the tendons in a rat's tail, and by Thomas Lewis on the haemolymphatic glands. And these achievements, by themselves, would have given little ground for expecting that their respective authors would later make such outstanding contributions to medical knowledge as Jenner's vaccination against small-pox, Waller's law governing the degeneration following nerve section, the discoveries by which Koch provided so much of the foundations of bacteriology, Horsley's work on the surgery and the functions of the brain, or Lewis's detailed elucidation of the origin and course of the heart-beat, in the higher vertebrates and in man. In any one of these cases, a contemporary qualified to judge would, indeed, have recognized the early signs of a notable faculty for keen and accurate observation, or, perhaps, of the ingenuity required to contrive the conditions for making it; but he could certainly not yet have found any reason for predicting the dimensions, still less the special direction, of the mature achievement which was to come.

It might be thought that Professor Gibson had rather restricted his opportunity, by confining his examples to discoveries made by students of medicine in particular; but I should be inclined to doubt the validity of any such suggestion. For it could be claimed, on the other hand, that the course of study for a medical career, lasting in so many cases for years after a primary, non-medical graduation, has enabled him very materially to extend the scope of his search, for discoveries by men who could still be classed as medical undergraduates. It should further be borne in mind that, until well into the nineteenth century, the opportunity, for the study of the experimental and observational sciences in general, was most often obtained in meeting the preclinical requirements of a medical course. It is no matter for surprise, accordingly, to find striking examples of men who were to become eminent figures, either in Chemistry or in Medicine, who gave early evidence of their powers by making chemical discoveries, even of fundamental importance, while they were still students of medicine. We read of Joseph Black, for instance, who was to become Professor of Medicine and Chemistry in the University of Glasgow, that his discovery of carbon dioxide, which he called "fixed air" —a discovery which, as Professor Gibson comments, "sounded the death knell of the traditional phlogiston theory"—was made while he was still an undergraduate student of medicine, and was described, indeed, in his graduation thesis; while Black's pupil, Daniel Rutherford, who was to become recognized as one of the founders of the Medical School at Edinburgh, where he was to be President of the Royal College of Physicians, was similarly in the undergraduate stage of his medical course when he discovered the residual, inert constituent of air, which he called "mephitic air," and which is now known as nitrogen, and which he also first described in his graduation thesis.

I feel that I must stand firmly against the temptation to quote further examples from Professor Gibson's fascinating collection. It is to be hoped that his book will become widely known and read, especially by the medical students of today, and by those who succeed them in the years ahead. It certainly ought to give them the sense of a more lively contact with a kind of mental discipline which they will essentially need at the bedside, or in the consulting-room, as well as in the laboratory. It may be hoped that many students will respond to its inspiration by finding, in spite of all difficulties and preoccupations, the opportunity for a personal experience of the eager pursuit of an enquiry, and of the joy which may come from discovery, or only, perhaps, from expecting it; for, here as elsewhere, it may often be true that "it is better to travel hopefully than to arrive."

H.H.D.

Introduction

THIS VOLUME treats of the contributions to science made by medical students of the past four centuries. None of the group is alive today. It is felt that in order to avoid invidious distinctions the living should not be discussed in the present volume. Nor would it be advisable to do so in the compass of one volume, so great would the number of individuals become. Large as the present list of undergraduate discoverers may seem it is undoubtedly but a fraction of those who will eventually be unearthed. The author must plead that the rigours of a medical researcher's and consultant's life have made a more thorough search impractical at this moment.

"Why, then," it may be asked, "should a possibly incomplete study be presented at all?" It is felt that sufficient material has been brought together to permit an appraisal of the rôle of medical students in the advancement of knowledge, past and future. At a time of major crisis in higher education, through which many countries are passing, it may be advisable to take a retrospective glance into the lives of these students of medicine. The findings may be applicable to other fields of professional education, but even by themselves, they may be sufficiently interesting to stimulate young minds to independent effort and hard thinking. This book might also stimulate teachers and researchers in our universities to give youthful minds entrusted to their tuition every opportunity to develop and to contribute. It is to be hoped that research grants committees, foundations and governments may come to view our undergraduate enquirers as a vital part of our human resources. Their misemployment today during their "vacations" as unskilled labourers must soon come to be recognized as shortsighted. Possibly quite soon we shall be able to say to our students, with John Masefield:

> Adventure on, for from the tiniest clue
> Has come whatever worth man ever knew;
> The next to lighten all men may be you.

A word of explanation may be in order concerning the term "medical student." A true undergraduate is meant—one who has yet to "qualify" as a physician entitled to practise his profession. Some, such as Galileo and Davy, never completed medicine. Some had already another calling—as Morton had in dentistry, and Pierre Marie had in law—but they were medical undergraduates when they made their first scientific contribution.

The grouping of the students according to fields of endeavour had to be arbitrary at times, but within chapters an attempt has been made at a chronological treatment. Illustrations have been included which may demonstrate the early works or the youthful features of the students concerned.

It is a pleasure to record the author's gratitude for assistance and inspiration received from many colleagues including Osler's Librarian, Dr. W. W. Francis, and his successor, Dr. Lloyd Stevenson, Dr. John F. Fulton and his staff at Yale University, Dr. Chauncey Leake and his staff at the University of Texas, Dr. Paul D. White, Dr. H. E. Rawlinson, Dr. S. E. C. Turvey, the late A. T. Rasmussen, Dr. Myron Weaver, and librarians in many parts of the world. My secretary, Miss Susan Calthrop and my wife have aided in innumerable ways with the manuscript and bibliography.

The doyen of medical researchers, Sir Henry Dale, O.M., has been kind enough to write a foreword. For his continued interest in this form of medical history, I am most grateful.

W. C. G.

Contents

List of Illustrations

YOUNG ENDEAVOUR

Chapter I

Anaesthesia

FROM THE synthesis of ether in 1540 by the German medical student Valerius Cordus to its introduction into surgical anaesthesia by W. T. G. Morton in 1846 there runs a well-nigh incredible story of opportunities missed by a hair's breadth, and of a succession of medical undergraduates whose contributions kept up a thread of continuity in this unusual tale.

The first of these undergraduates, Valerius Cordus, was born in 1515 into a family where a concern for education and botany was uppermost. His father [Euricius] came from Hessian peasant stock and graduated in ancient languages and philology at the University of Erfurth, ten years after Martin Luther. With the Reformation making for widespread civil and ecclesiastical disturbances, Euricius Cordus decided to study medicine as a safer calling than some others. He was eventually made Professor of Medicine at Marburg in 1527.

From his father Valerius learned languages, botany and the fundamentals of materia medica. At the age of sixteen he enrolled at the University of Wittemberg in medicine. He often visited his uncle, Joachim Ralla, an apothecary living in Leipzig, and it was there that Valerius Cordus synthesized ether by distilling together "sour oil of vitriol" (sulphuric acid) with "very biting wine" (alcohol). His description of the process in chemical terms is remarkable, and is well illustrated by sketches.

Cordus recorded some interesting things about ether, even if he wrote nothing about its anaesthetic properties. This *oleum dulci vitrioli*, as he called it, he knew to be a solvent of great volatility, which, he wrote, "may be used in pleurisy, peripneumonia and hacking cough to draw from the lungs pus and mucus. . . . It heals an ulcerated urinary bladder." He added, probably from sad experience, "It must be carefully observed, however, for only a little is got from a pound of sour oil of vitriol, and because . . . it easily evaporates."

It is of incidental interest that Cordus, as a medical student aged nineteen, compiled a pharmacopoeia for cities in Saxony and at age twenty he wrote one for Nuremberg, which was eventually published by the Senate of the city in 1546; it ran through thirty-five editions and eight translations.

Cordus is known today chiefly as a founder of modern botany. While still in his teens he set out to remedy the situation in which German botanists found themselves. The textbooks in use were largely repetitions of the discoveries made by Theophrastus, Dioscorides and Pliny, of the plants known around the Mediterranean basin. Cordus showed that the German alpine and forest lands would yield large numbers of new species if studied systematically. He described over five hundred such species in Germany and Italy. It was in the pursuit of this work in 1544 that he contracted a fever in the malarial marshes of the southern Italian coast, and died at the age of twenty-nine. Haller, himself a student contributor, said of Cordus that he was "the first to teach man to cease from dependence upon the poor description of the ancients and to describe plants anew from Nature." The early apprenticeship served in medicine undoubtedly enabled Cordus to make the broad generalizations and the classifications of plant life which so distinguished his contributions to science.

Of his work on ether Chauncey Leake has written: "There is no doubt that Valerius Cordus gave the first clear account of the synthesis of ether from sulphuric acid and alcohol. This account is so carefully written, and the details so completely given, that it stamps Valerius as among the first to make the transition from the mystical aims of alchemy to the rational ends of chemistry."

The fate of Cordus' ether is not clearly known, but it is of interest that Paracelcus, who died in 1541, had heard of ether, calling it by the name "sulphur." He wrote: "It possesses an agreeable taste; even chickens will eat it, whereupon they sleep for a moderately long time, and re-awake without having been injured. There is no other evidence of the action of this sulphur than that in diseases which are treated by allaying the pain, it cures all of the disorders, relieves all of the pains."

This lead which, in retrospect, we consider remarkable in its import, was not followed up to any useful degree, for approximately three hundred years. A Liverpool surgeon, Matthew Turner, used linen sponges soaked in ether and applied to the nose to relieve severe headache in 1743. Lavoisier thought ether a sound remedy for migraine.

The 19-year old medical student, Humphry Davy, is the next to enter the picture. He is regarded by some as the discoverer of surgical anaesthesia. He was apprenticed in medicine to John Bingham Borlase of Penzance, Cornwall, a year after his father's death. His boyhood had been more than usually full of broad scientific and cultural interests, and he took in his stride history, the making of gun powder, the smelting of tin from the local mines, fishing, writing poems and plays, acting, mineralizing, and chemical experimentation. His schooling in Cornwall was completed at Truro, the home of William Osler's family.

Davy was a precocious and eclectic genius. He tried to discover whether the plants of the ocean regulated the salinity of the sea as land plants did that of the soil. He made the most of his limited resources. When a French ship was wrecked on the coast near Penzance, Davy secured some syringes from the medical chest washed ashore. With these he made a rudimentary air pump and evacuated a large glass bell jar beneath which he placed some ice and a clockwork motor. The heat generated by the motor melted the ice in proportion to the "work done"—the origin of Davy's contribution on "The fusion of ice by friction."

It is related that while swinging on the gate of Dr. Borlase's

No uniformity in life is found:—
In ev'ry scene varieties abound;
And inconsistency still marks the plan
Of that immortal noble being, Man.
As changeful as the April's morning skies,
His feeling and his sentiments arise;
And nature to his wond'rous frame has given
The mingled elements of earth and heaven.
In diff'rent climes and ages, still we find
The same events for diff'rent ends design'd:
And the same passion diff'rent minds can move
To thoughts of sadness or to acts of love.
  Hence Genius draws his novel copious store;
And hence the new creations we adore:
And hence the scenic art's undying skill
Submits our feeling to its potent will;
From common accidents and common themes
Awakens rapture and poetic dreams;
And, in the trodden path of life, pursues
Some object cloth'd in Fancy's loveliest hues—"

HUMPHRY DAVY.

(From his Prologue written for *The Honey Moon* produced at Drury Lane, 30 January, 1805.)

house in Penzance, Davy was "discovered" by Mr. Davies Gilbert, a very learned man, who lost no time in offering the use of his library to the young medical apprentice. Soon there followed an invitation to use the chemical laboratory of a Doctor Edwards who lived in the district, and who later lectured in Chemistry at St. Bartholomew's Hospital.

Davy had set his heart on graduation in medicine from Edinburgh, but when Davies Gilbert proposed his name to Professor Beddoes as a researcher for the latter's Pneumatic Institution in Bristol, the Edinburgh dream was deferred, though never forgotten. Dr. Borlase, believing in Davy's future, released him from his apprenticeship, and in 1798 Davy arrived in Bristol.

The Pneumatic Institution, one of Joseph Priestley's concepts, was a remarkable place—a forerunner of our modern "day hospital"—in which eighty non-resident cases were treated. Thomas Beddoes, who possessed a medical degree from Oxford, was keen to explore the medicinal uses to which gases could be put. He had met Lavoisier in Paris, he had worked with Cullen in Edinburgh, and, of especial interest here, he had, as an undergraduate, translated Spallanzani's *Dissertations on Natural History*. Beddoes was anathema to Tory Bristol, for he associated with such advanced thinkers as Robert Southey and Samuel Taylor Coleridge, Wedgwood, and Joseph Priestley's son. This fact must be kept in mind in what follows.

By 1799 Davy was experimenting with nitrous oxide, using instruments made for him by James Watt. He recorded on April 10th the results of breathing purified nitrous oxide which "made me dance about the laboratory as a madman." He noted the changes in sensation and in motor power from inhaling too much of the gas. Headaches induced by the rapid ingestion of large amounts of wine could be relieved by nitrous oxide. A Mr. Clayfield lost consciousness from deep inhalations of it.

In July of 1799 Davy wrote: "In one instance, when I had headache from indigestion, it was immediately removed by the effects of a large dose of the gas, though it afterwards returned, but with much less violence. In a second instance, a slighter degree of headache was wholly removed by two doses of gas.

"The power of the immediate operation of the gas in re-

"Like the tumultuous billows of the sea
Succeed the generations of mankind;
Some in oblivious silence pass away,
And leave no vestige of their lives behind.

Others, like those proud waves which beat the shore,
A loud and momentary murmur raise;
But soon their transient glories are no more.
No future ages echo with their praise.

Like yon proud rock, amidst the sea of time,
Superior, scorning all the billows' rage,
The living Sons of Genius stand sublime,
The immortal children of another age.

For those exist whose pure ethereal minds,
Imbibing portions of celestial day,
Scorn all terrestrial cares, all mean designs,
As bright-eyed eagles scorn the lunar ray.

Theirs is the glory of a lasting name,
The meed of Genius, and her living fire;
Theirs is the laurel of eternal fame,
And theirs the sweetness of the muse's lyre."

From *The Sons of Genius*, by HUMPHRY DAVY.

moving intense physical pain, I had a very good opportunity of ascertaining.

"In cutting one of the unlucky teeth called *dentes sapientiae*, I experienced an extensive inflammation of the gum, accompanied with great pain, which equally destroyed the power to repose, and of consistent action.

"On the day when the inflammation was most troublesome, I breathed three large doses of nitrous oxide. The pain always diminished after the first four or five inspirations."

In 1800 came the publication of Humphry Davy's classic *Researches, Chemical and Philosophical, Chiefly Concerning Nitrous Oxide* with the immortal paragraph on page 556: "As nitrous oxide in its extensive operation appears capable of destroying physical pain, it may probably be used with advantage during surgical operations in which no great effusion of blood takes place." Unfortunately no one read as far as page 556, or understood this proclamation of the surgical anaesthetic value of nitrous oxide.

Before leaving Davy we should recall the fact that at the age of sixteen in Cornwall he had drawn up a remarkable plan of study for himself. As late as 1811 he was keeping terms at Cambridge, hoping to graduate in medicine.

It was not long before nitrous oxide's properties became well known across the Atlantic, and in 1808 we find an undergraduate at the University of Pennsylvania writing in his thesis that, "The effect of breathing nitrous oxyd" was "the only genteel way of getting drunk." Davy's views and some of his expressions were used in this student's essay.

The poet, Robert Southey, wrote of nitrous oxide: "The atmosphere of the highest of all possible heavens must be composed of this gas." This appeared in a Hartford, Connecticut, newspaper advertising one of a series of lectures by a man named Colton. A dentist of that town, Horace Wells, attended a Colton lecture where he saw a man gash his knee on some furniture while under the influence of nitrous oxide, without feeling any pain. Wells tried the gas on himself, on cases in his dental surgery, and eventually demonstrated it, though unsuccessfully, at the Massachusetts General Hospital. Wells' one-time partner in dentistry, William

"I weigh my words when I say that if the nation could purchase a potential Watt, or Davy, or Faraday, at the cost of £100,000 down, he would be dirt-cheap at the money. It is a mere commonplace and everyday piece of knowledge that what these men did has produced untold millions of wealth in the narrowest economic sense of the word."

—Thomas Huxley, 1877.

". . . . . . I trust that those amongst us who are so fortunate as to kindle the light of new discoveries will use them not for the purpose of dazzling the organs of our intellectual vision but rather to enlighten us, by showing objects in their true form and colors; that our philosophers will attach no importance to hypotheses except as leading to the research after facts so as to be able to discard or adopt them at pleasure treating them rather as parts of the scaffolding of the building of science."

Sir Humphry Davy to Fellows of the Royal Society in 1820.

T. G. Morton, became so interested in nitrous oxide anaesthesia that he decided to take a medical training, and entered the office of Dr. Charles T. Jackson in Boston, and later Harvard Medical School. Jackson, as an undergraduate, had read Humphry Davy's *Researches.*

As a medical student and a busy dental practitioner, Morton began to explore ether as a potential anaesthetic agent, steering away from nitrous oxide, which, in Horace Wells' hands, had proven fatal in one case. Morton began cautiously with experiments on goldfish, puppies, worms and caterpillars! One of his dogs upset a bottle of ether and this the student Morton soaked up in a handkerchief, which, when held to his face, caused a definite change in sensibility to pain.*

Jackson advised his student to try pure sulphuric ether, instead of chloric ether, and immediately Morton's results improved. He anaesthetized himself for a period of seven to eight minutes and made an uneventful recovery. Then he induced two dental students, Thomas Spear and William Leavitt, to submit to trials of ether, and on September 30, 1846, Morton administered this substance to Eben Frost in the course of a dental extraction.

Within a week Morton approached his surgical teacher at the Massachusetts General Hospital, John Collins Warren, a senior surgeon, aged 68, who had years before investigated all possible methods of anaesthesia, including hypnotism. Morton was granted permission to demonstrate his method of ether anaesthesia on October 16, 1846—in the same amphitheatre in which the ill-fated Wells had failed in an attempt to prove the value of nitrous oxide.

The story of Morton's successful demonstration is too well-known to require repetition here. Suffice it to say that his success was based on two and a half years of hard work as a medical student, struggling to keep up his studies and his dental practice while still experimenting with ether. That he was not alone in this type of adventure is shown by the fact that William E. Clarke,

* Prior to his graduation in Philadelphia in 1839 Crawford Long (1815-1878) had inhaled ether along with his medical student friends behind locked doors in their Quaker boarding house! His personal experience induced him to try it as an anaesthetic in 1842 in Georgia.

a medical student from Rochester, New York, registered at the Berkshire Medical College, was in 1841 experimenting with ether on his classmates. In January 1842, in Rochester, he gave ether to a Miss Hobbie while Dr. Elijah Pope, a dentist, removed a tooth without causing pain of any kind. This use of ether occurred two months prior to the now-famous surgical operation by Crawford Long in Georgia in March 1842.

Thus, the forerunners in the field of surgical anaesthesia are clearly seen to be medical students, from Cordus to Morton. Their contributions vary in approach and emphasis, but all have assisted in putting together the mosaic of modern anaesthesia.

→

PLATE 1

(a) Sketch by the undergraduate Valerius Cordus of the apparatus he used in synthesizing ether. From: *Isis,* 7:14-24, 1925. Courtesy of Chauncey Leake.

(b) Valerius Cordus' student *Dispensatorium* published by the Nuremberg Senate. Courtesy of the National Library of Medicine, Cleveland.

(c) Robert Watt, M.D. (1774-1819), author of the *Bibliotheca Britannica.* Courtesy of Dr. Francesco Cordasco, Long Island University.

(d) John Shaw Billings in Civil War surgeon's uniform, at the age of twenty-five. From: Fulton, J. F.: *The Great Medical Bibliographers,* Philadelphia, 1951. Courtesy of the University of Pennsylvania Press.

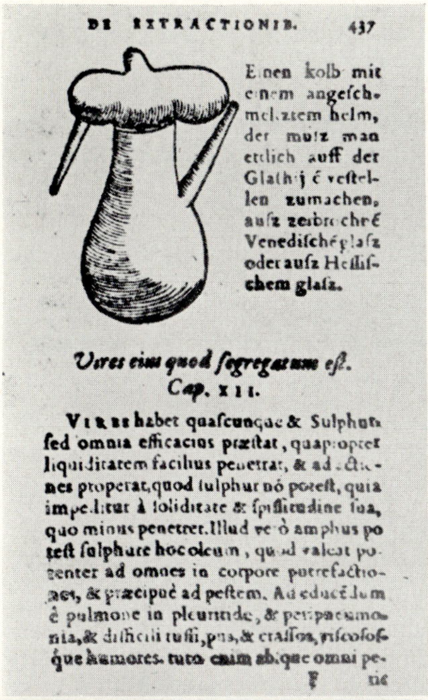

DE EXTRACTIONIB. 437

Einen kolb mit einem angeschmelztem helm, der mutz man etlich auff der Glathij e vestellen zumachen, ausz zerbrochne Venedischéglasz oder ausz Hessischem glasz.

Vires eius quod segregatum est.
Cap. XII.

VIRES habet quascunque & Sulphur, sed omnia efficacius præstat, quapropter liquiditatem facilius penetrat, & ad actiones properat, quod sulphur nó potest, quia impeditur à soliditate & spissitudine sua, quo minus penetret. Illud veró amplius potest sulphure hoc oleum, quod valeat potenter ad omnes in corpore putrefactiones, & præcipué ad pestem. Ad educẽdum é pulmone in pleuritide, & peripneumonia, & difficili tussi, pus, & crassos, viscososque humores. tuto enim absque omni pe-

F tie

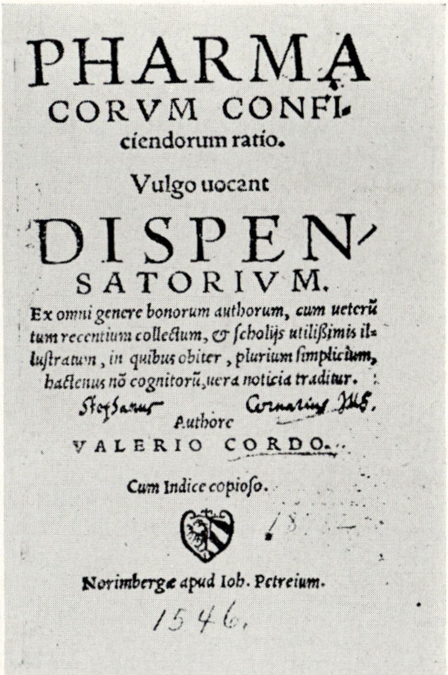

PHARMACORVM CONFIciendorum ratio.

Vulgo uocant

DISPENSATORIVM.

Ex omni genere bonorum authorum, cum ueterũ tum recentium collectum, & scholijs utilißimis illustratum, in quibus obiter, plurium simplicium, hactenus nõ cognitorũ, uera noticia traditur.

Authore

VALERIO CORDO.

Cum Indice copioso.

Norimbergæ apud Ioh. Petreium.

1546.

Title-page of the first edition of the DISPENSATORIUM of VALERIUS CORDUS. From the Library of the Surgeon-General's Office. Note date penciled in.

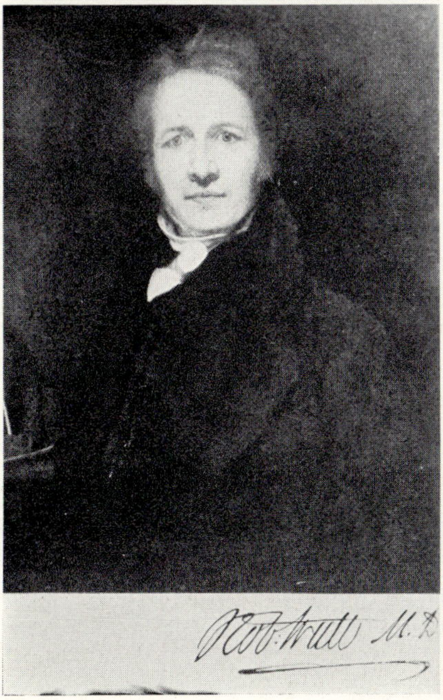

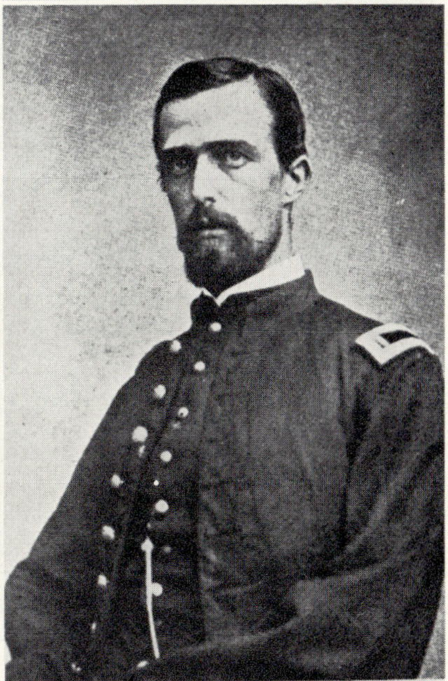

John Shaw Billings at age of twenty-five

Chapter II

Anatomy

Andreas Vesalius (1514-1564)

MODERN MEDICINE owes much to Andreas Vesalius who gave us the first text on human anatomy since the Christian era began. His contribution stands with that of William Harvey in the magnitude of its influence on science.

Vesalius was born in 1514 in Brussels, of German stock, by name Wesel, and of Dutch ancestors from Nimwegen. His mother, Isabella Crabbe, was English. His father was court pharmacist to King Charles V, whom he accompanied on journeys throughout his vast kingdom. His grandfather was a court physician, who wrote a commentary on Rhazes. His great-grandfather was physician to Emperor Maximilian's wife. His great-great-grandfather was also a physician and wrote a discourse on the works of Avicenna. It is little wonder, then, that our subject wrote a book of commentaries also, on the Ninth Book of Rhazes, as his graduation dissertation. Vesalius was still in the medieval tradition of Arabic medicine, but he was to make his mark as a humanist, a student of Galen, before he became the first modern anatomist himself. He thus represents all three stages in his own person.

As a comparatively young boy Andreas showed an interest in

anatomy, dissecting rats, cats and dogs, and in studying a skeleton retrieved from a gallows not far from his home. His preliminary studies in the classics were made at Louvain under Johann Guenther of Andernach, who was later to be his teacher of anatomy in Paris.

As a medical student in Paris Vesalius relied on the Cemetery of the Innocents at Montfaucon for a supply of bones. He tells of having to compete for these bones with vicious dogs at times! His other outstanding teacher in Paris was Jacobus Sylvius—later to be his severest critic.

It is known that Vesalius was an extremely hard worker in his student days in Paris. Guinterius Andernacus wrote of Vesalius' assistance in a study of the asymmetrical position of the seminal veins: "It was only recently found with the help of Andreas Vesalius, son of the Emperor's pharmacist—a young man, by Jove, of great promise, possessing a singular knowledge of medicine, erudite in both languages [Latin and Greek] and most skilled in dissecting bodies—after extensive research in the parts of the human body." *

Vesalius came to Paris already knowing considerable *human* anatomy. His knowledge was superimposed upon the emotional background of a potential rebel—and it was not long before he was in full revolt against what he saw in Paris, as his words suggest:

> The lecturers are perched up in a pulpit like jackdaws, and arrogantly prate about things they have never tried, but have committed to memory from the books of others, or placed in written form before their eyes. The dissectors are so ignorant of language that they are unable to explain their dissections to the onlookers, and merely botch what they are supposed to exhibit in accordance with the instructions of the physician, who never applies his hand to the dissection, but contemptuously steers the ship out of the manual, as the saying goes. Thus everything is wrongly

* Guinterius, a liberal Catholic, taught another great contributor, Michael Servetus, who discovered the lesser circulation from the right to the left heart through the lungs which he first described in *Restitutio Christianismi* (1553). Servetus, at the age of twenty, began publishing his supposedly heretical works for which he was burned at the stake by John Calvin, in 1553. Guinterius described Servetus as "a man who would be an ornament of any branch of letters, and who is second to none in the Galenical doctrine."

> taught, days are wasted in absurd questions, and in the confusion less is offered to the onlooker than a butcher in his stall could teach a doctor.
>
> Except for eight muscles of the abdomen, disgracefully mangled and in the wrong order, no one . . . ever demonstrated to me any single muscle, or any single bone, much less the network of nerves, veins and arteries.

It is little wonder that after witnessing two incompetent dissections, Vesalius should jump into the third one—done on a dog—to show his fellow students the true and beautiful "fabric of the body," to be followed by many more such demonstrations.

In 1536, with war brewing, he returned to his home in Louvain to serve in the army. He carried on further anatomizing and during 1537 published his graduation dissertation, probably already completed in Paris, on Rhazes, *De singularum corporis partium affectuum curatione*. (It was printed in Louvain by his friend of Paris days, Rutger Resch, and reprinted in Basel by Robert Winter.) This he dedicated to his friend and patron Nicolaus Florenas, physician to the Emperor. With the same spiritual broom used on Galen, he began his re-edition of Rhazes, "cleansed of errors and clothed in elegant Latin style." One is reminded of the service performed somewhat earlier by another purgative spirit, Lorenzo Valla, in his "Elegant Latin Language" (1476).*

In this graduation thesis Vesalius stated his objective thus:

> . . . I have started to revise the translation of Rhazes, both in order to liberate other candidates of medicine from immense labour, and to enable the author himself to reach men's hands henceforth cleansed of all barbarian names of medicaments unrecognizable to Latin ears, and with his entire mode of expression changed for the better; so that what was heretofore squalid and coarse and too obscure to be intelligible, will now be brightened, as far as possible, and will require the least exertion from the reader.

Foreshadowing later events and writings Vesalius concludes with an exhortation to his patron:

* The frauds in translation uncovered by Valla in his beautifully printed book (see Sherrington copy in University of British Columbia Library) were of the magnitude of the half truths in Galen uncovered by Vesalius.

I ask you, then, to defend this prelude of my studies with serene and smooth brow against quibblers, and to regard with benignity whatever you deem in it to be worthy, until such time as I shall produce something greater and more suitable to your excellent learning. Farewell, ornament of all physicians; may you help our august Emperor Charles, whom at present the Christian World cannot afford to lose, to long and happy life.

In the same year (1537) Vesalius sought the liberal atmosphere of Padua, graduating as a Doctor of Medicine there on December 5th, and being made Professor the following day! Within four months, with the help of Calcar, a Belgian pupil of Titian, he published six *Tabulae Anatomicae* for his students. In order to provide them with an interim textbook he personally re-edited Guinterius' *Institutiones Anatomicae*, (a commentary on Galen) and published it in May, 1538, only six months after taking up his Chair.

Vesalius' publications now began to pyramid in a truly amazing manner. In 1539, at the age of 25, he published his *Epistola Docens* on venesection, and turned then to Galen's texts, three volumes of which he edited for the Venetian publishers Giunta.* In 1540, convinced that he must put down a record of his own findings in human dissections he started to write his 700-page *De Fabrica Humani Corporis*, which he completed in August of 1542. His publishing did not prevent his teaching from human dissections. It is interesting to note that what Vesalius was doing for students at the dissecting table, his Paduan pupil, Montanus, was to do eventually for medical student-teaching at the bedside.

Some historians have made much of Vesalius' exit from Padua under a storm of criticism, soon after the publication of the *Fabrica*, and of his twenty-year period at the Spanish court of the marauding Charles V and his son Phillip II. Vesalius died on the Island of Zante in Greece while returning from a pilgrimage to Jerusalem, at the age of fifty.

As a letter written to his successor Fallopius at Padua suggests,

* Vesalius refers to Galen later as "after Hippocrates the prince of medicine," and "easily the foremost among the teachers of anatomy."

"Furthermore, these pernicious men are not above speaking slander, if they notice any one who knows things of which they are ignorant, they admit that he is well versed in those subjects but deny that he is a physician. . . . Just as if a man should be considered a physician only when he is nothing else, or as if unlimited diligence in any of the branches of study subservient to medicine would impair one's knowledge of the art itself. . . . The physicians who advance this opinion are those with no knowledge of medicine except for some drugs that cleanse the bowels, and syrups that cause the evacuation of humours."

—Vesalius, *Epistola Chynae.*

Vesalius, after an absence of seventeen years, still longed for the academic life—"that most delightful life, which, teaching anatomy, I passed in Italy, the true nurse of intellects . . . I look forward to see the ornaments of our science continue to bud forth in the school from which I was while yet a youngster dragged away to the dull routine of medical practice and to the worries of continual journeys."

But surely Vesalius' accomplishments merit more attention than do the unhappy twenty years of gloom which his too-rash decision to leave Padua brought on. (No more complete isolation from his old subject can be imagined than that behind the Pyrenees, where, he complained, he could not even obtain a skull to anatomize.)

Vesalius was also a physiologist. He removed the spleen in an animal, with no ill-effects (just as Christopher Wren was to do a century later). Vesalius cut the recurrent laryngeal nerve producing aphonia or loss of voice as Galen had done before him. He sliced living muscle tissue in the long axis of the fibres and found little or no disability. He pierced the thoracic wall of animals and kept them alive by artificial respiration through a bellows.

Vesalius' pupil and successor, Fallopius, taught Fabricius, who, in turn, taught William Harvey at Padua. Thus we see the passing on of the spirit of enquiry from an anatomist interested in physiology to a physiologist who finally made sense of the anatomy of the heart and circulation. One is reminded of the words of Jean Fernel (1497-1557): "Anatomy is to physiology as geography is to history—it gives the setting of the events."

We lightly speak of the pen changing the world more effectually than the sword, and yet when we contemplate the year 1543 we cannot but believe that it is so. In that year the writings of two physicians shook the world of thought. These were the posthumous astronomical work of Copernicus, *De Revolutionibus Orbium Coelestium*, and *De Humani Corporis Fabrica* of Vesalius.

Osler sums it up well when he says: "In itself, for what it contains but still more for what it did, the 'Humani Corporis Fabrica' is one of the great books of the world, with which, in the literature of Medicine only the 'De motu cordis' of Harvey is to be compared. . . . The 'Fabrica' remains a monument of human effort, one of the greatest in the history of our profession."

Lorenzo Bellini (1643-1704)

Galileo, during his time at Pisa, numbered among his associates such men as the histologist Malpighi and the physicist Borelli. The latter was one of the first to attempt purely physical explanations for the microscopic workings of the body organs. Associated with him in this was a medical student, Lorenzo Bellini, whose name is still applied to the "straight tubules" of the kidney which conduct the newly formed urine to the apex of the "pyramids of Malpighi," on its way to the ureter and the bladder.

In 1662, the 19-year old Bellini was anatomizing a deer, sent to Borelli by the Duke of Tuscany, when he discovered the "straight tubules." Although the great anatomist, Eustachius, after whom is named the Eustachian tube of the ear, had mentioned minute tubules in the kidney, it remained for the alert Bellini to grasp their nature and meaning clearly. It is likely, moreover, that a pupil of the physicist Borelli should propose a purely physical theory to account for the separation of the urine from the large amount of blood which coursed through the kidneys—a volume of blood now known to be as much as one thousand litres per day.

Bellini pictured the "serous" or fluid part of the blood giving rise to the urine by some sort of separation within the peripheral tissue of the kidney, and then continuing through the channels, already mentioned, to the bladder. The blood corpuscles, on the other hand, remained in the blood vessels and left the kidney by the renal veins. The degree of separation of these elements depended upon the comparative sizes of the urine-bearing tubules and the veins leaving the kidney.

Bellini could see no cause to introduce any chemical theory into the discussion and wrote: "Inside the body changes of mechanical pressure suffice to explain all that takes place. A gland is simply a closed vessel with extremely small perforations of different shape and size. . . . There is not the slightest necessity for complicating the matter with ferments."

It is not surprising that this eminent pupil of Borelli should become Professor of Anatomy at Pisa and eventually physician to Cosimo III at Florence. He wrote *De Urinis et pulsibus, de missione sanguinis, de febribus, de morbis capitis, et pectoris*, published in Frankfurt and Leipzig in 1695, and described calcification of the coronary arteries. Bellini's name is associated in our minds today, however, with his undergraduate contribution on the kidney tubules, *Exercitatio anatomica de structura Et usu renum*, published in Florence in 1662.

Johann Hamm (Hamen) (1650-1723)

Next in our chronology we encounter Johann Hamm (Hamen) from Arnheim in Holland. He was, as a medical student, working with Anthony van Leeuwenhoek in Leyden when in 1674 he discovered the structure of human spermatozoa under his microscope. Leeuwenhoek confirmed the discovery, extended the observation to other animals, and then sent the work to the Royal Society of London in one of his 375 communications to that body. In Leeuwenhoek's quaint phraseology the sperms became "little men" and "little women." Parenthetically it may be noted that Leeuwenhoek did not begin publishing until the age of 41, but he continued to work and to write till the end of his life, 50 years later!

Johann Friedrich Meckel (1724-1774)

In the year after Hamm's death Johann Friedrich Meckel was born in Wetzlar. Thus began that distinguished line of Prussian anatomists which was to number his son Phillip (1756-1803), Professor of Anatomy at Halle, two grandsons, Johann Friedrich (1781-1833) called "the younger," and known as "the German Cuvier," and August Albrecht (1790-1829), Professor of Anatomy at Berne.

Johann Friedrich Meckel, "the elder," wrote his graduation thesis *De quinto pare nervorum cerebri* at the age of twenty-four, describing the ganglion which still bears his name. Phillip graduated in Strasbourg in 1777 with a dissertation of great merit on the internal ear, *De labyrinthi auris contentis.*

The "younger" Meckel is known for his work on "Meckel's diverticulum" but he was also to bring to public notice the classical texts of embryology by Caspar Friedrich Wolff (1733-

1794), by translating them into German. Wolff, known to every student for the "Wolffian body" or primitive kidney, wrote the first of his revolutionary doctrines in his graduation thesis *Theoria Generationis* in 1759. His view, like Harvey's, was that the embryo develops gradually, and is not a mere prefabricated "creature in miniature" awaiting release from the ovary. Few have rivalled the originality of thought displayed by this master observer and "father of embryology."

Henry Gray (1827-1861)

Gray's *Anatomy* is known the world over. Strangely, little is known about Gray. He was born in 1827. His father is said to have been the private messenger to George IV and to William IV. On May 6, 1845, Henry Gray entered St. George's Hospital Medical School in London as a "perpetual student."

It is recorded that Gray was "a most painstaking and methodical worker, and one who learnt his anatomy by the slow but invaluable method of making dissections for himself." We know that while he was a student he prepared an essay of 341 pages which won the Triennial Prize of the Royal College of Surgeons in 1848, the year of his qualifying examinations for the M.R.C.S. His subject was *The Origin, Connection and Distribution of the Nerves of the Human Eye and its Appendages*, illustrated by Comparative Dissections of the Eye of other Vertebrate Animals. According to Miss Jessie Dobson, Recorder of the Royal College of Surgeons and an able historian, "It contains several drawings of high merit, presumably his own work, and the whole thing gives evidence of his enthusiastic and painstaking industry."

This student dissertation is probably without parallel as a comprehensive survey of the phylogeny of the nervous structures associated with vision and eye movements. After dealing with the visual apparatus of the cuttle fish and the octopus he details the arrangements in fish, reptiles and birds. On page 65 he starts on the mammals, and includes the stag, the horse, and the porpoise. The anatomy of the trigeminal and facial nerves is covered, together with the distribution of the sympathetic nerves. Then he launches into a 257-page treatise on the structures associated with vision in the human.

Gray studied both the gross and microscopic structures involved in vision, in rotating the eye-ball, in closing the eyelids, in regulating the "nutrition" of the eye, in controlling the secretion of tears and in regulating the size of the pupil and the curvature of the lens. He went to the heart of things and pursued the "orbital nerves" back to their origin within the medulla oblongata. From his own dissections and from preparations which he studied at the Museum of the Royal College of Surgeons, Gray collected the material for this amazing work.

Qualifying in 1848, he became a demonstrator in anatomy at St. George's Hospital, Curator of the Museum and eventually lecturer in anatomy. In 1850 he carried his earlier work further and wrote a paper on the development of the retina and optic nerve, and of the membranous labyrinth of the ear and the auditory nerve. In 1852 he published a paper on the development of the ductless or inwardly secreting glands of the chick, and a year later described a remarkable ovarian cyst which contained brain tissue. At the age of twenty-five he was made a Fellow of the Royal Society. In the same year he was awarded the Astley Cooper Prize of 300 guineas for a dissertation: "On the Structure and Use of the Spleen."

Gray's monumental *Anatomy, Descriptive and Surgical* was published in 1858, when he was thirty-two. It was a book of 750 pages. Its 363 illustrations were made with the help of Dr. Vandyke Carter, a friend "skilled in illustration." The book was so popular that a second edition was required in 1860.

Gray died at the age of thirty-four of smallpox contracted from a nephew whom he was attending. It should not be imagined that Henry Gray's scientific work ceased when he became the author of a great textbook. At the time of his death he was working on a book on tumors.

Gray's undergraduate labours fitted him to produce the book which still bears his name and is still in daily use. Although a gifted dissector and illustrator, Gray repeatedy said that his book was but an extension of his teaching arm, and that he had written it for students who wanted to learn rather than for anatomists alone.

Frederick Oldfield Ward (1818-1877)

Frederick Ward was educated at Dr. Knox's School in Tonbridge up to the age of fifteen when he entered the Medical

School of King's College Hospital, London. He distinguished himself there, winning a medal in chemistry in 1835 and one in botany in 1837. At the age of twenty, and while still a medical student he published his *Human Osteology*, one of the most remarkable books in the long history of anatomy.

The volume was the size and shape of a small prayerbook, but what it lacked in size it made up in substance. The simplicity of its prose and illustrations is something rarely found in our expensive texts today.

In the preface Ward says that his little volume was the product "partly of researches in the museum and dissecting room, prosecuted at intervals during the last five years: partly of a careful perusal and comparison of the best English and foreign works on the subject." His aim, he said, was brevity. "But holding that true brevity consists not in expressing ideas in a small space but in conveying them in a short time, I have not thought it inconsistent with this design to dilate freely upon some obscure and difficult points which have been passed over in a few lines by previous writers. . . . Whatever contradictory statements came under my notice in the course of this comparison were noted down, and made the subject of careful research in several extensive anatomical collections . . . which afforded me the opportunity of comparing nearly two hundred specimens of each bone."

This Vesalian spirit went further. Ward tested the oft reported elasticity of the clavicle by hammering it longitudinally against a stone wall and observing its spring. He tested too the strength of the lateral condyle of the femur and found that each cubic inch could support "four hundred weight without sensible alteration."

"Ward's Triangle" in the neck of the femur, so familiar to radiologists today, was described on page 370 of his *Human Osteology* with accompanying figures, thus (see page 39): "The structure of the neck is shown at Fig. 1 in the subjoined diagram. It resembles in its mechanical principles a bracket of the kind represented in Fig 2 in which *a* is the principal support, and *b* a cross-piece tying *a* to the wall or column which sustains the whole. It is evident that the piece *a* contributed by its rigidty, and the piece *b* by its tenacity, to the support of the weight; in other

> words, that the weight tends to bend the former, and to stretch the latter. Referring to Figure 1 (in which the direction of the principal fibres is shown with fictitious distinctness, the cross filaments, etc., being purposely omitted) we find the pieces *a* and *b* of the bracket respectively represented by the sets of bony fibres marked *aa* and *bb*. The fibres aa are inclined columns supporting the epiphysis of the head *cc* and resting below upon the thick wall *d* of the neck. The transverse fibres *bb* decussate the columns *aa*, and tie them to the thin upper wall *e* of the neck, and to the arch-work *ff* of the upper extremity. The middle of this arch-work presents a column of more condensed tissue, indicated by the shaded portion *f* in the diagram: this results partly from the decussation of the convergent fibres, partly from the presence of several bony canals for the reception of nutrient vessels, that here descend vertically into the bone through orifices in the upper wall of the neck. The interval *g* (which obviously corresponds to the interval *g* between the parts *a* and *b* of the bracket, Fig. 2) is filled with a loose reticular tissue, presenting no determinate nor uniform arrangement." He described a like area in the calcaneum of the foot, still known as "Ward's triangle of the calcaneum."

A second edition of his book appeared in 1856 and a third in 1875. Ward died in St. George's Retreat Lunatic Asylum, near Lewes, in 1877. His life, after the propitious start we have seen, became one long series of legal and personal duels, with his friend Mowbray Morris, manager of *The Times*, and with tradesmen who infringed various patents which he had bought up. In fact, the course of his later life is reminiscent of that of William Morton of anaesthesia fame.

Ward wrote for *The Times* on public health matters, but took it into his head to offer to re-organize the newspaper for a consideration. In the same way he proposed to re-organize the sanitation and water supply of Great Britain under one board of control. He was actually appointed, on Lord Palmerston's recommendation, Commissioner of Sewers in London, and devised an all-inclusive drainage plan for London. His office was short-lived, however, and we can only speculate on the cause of his "enfeeblement," referred to in *Personal Recollections* by Sir John Simon, the Medical Officer of Health of London, and a classmate of Ward's at King's College.

Ward remains as a name in radiological anatomy, and, for us, the student author of a very remarkable little textbook.

Thomas Huxley (1825-1895)

The blissful calm of the Victorian era was shattered by two medical students and their theory of evolution. Charles Darwin and his "bulldog," Thomas Huxley, were to hold the stage in England for almost sixty years as they indoctrinated and divided the country.

Darwin entered upon medicine at Edinburgh but gave it up after two terms because some of the lectures were "incredibly dull." He then decided to study for the church but gave that up, ending by taking his B.A. at Cambridge. He sailed on the H.M.S. Beagle as naturalist to the expedition which lasted from 1831 to 1836. It was in that year, as he sought to classify the specimens brought back, that he made journal notes of his theory of evolution.

In the same year Thomas Huxley was moving from the school at Ealing where his father taught, in order to support his seven children, to Coventry where self-education became the order of things. At the age of twelve Thomas was lighting his candle early in the morning in order to read Hutton's *Geology*. His brother-in-law, Dr. Cooke of Coventry, early stimulated Thomas' interest in anatomy, and it is recorded that the young student contracted an infection while attending an autopsy. He read Sir William Hamilton's *Logic* and taught himself German.

Huxley at the age of 15 was keeping a journal and speculated on "what would become of things if their qualities were taken away." He noted down quotations from Goethe, and speculated on the origin of the colors in the sunset. His social conscience was maturing rapidly and he wrote: "I think now that it is against all the laws of justice to force men to support a church with whose opinions they cannot conscientiously agree. I wonder what will be my opinion ten years hence?" At least one bishop was to find out clearly what Huxley's views were to be, as we shall see presently.

Huxley spent some time in making a galvanic battery which would deposit carbon. He was forever experimenting with things electrical and wrote in his journal on January 30, 1842: "I have for some time been pondering over a classification of knowledge" —at age sixteen! By then he was apprenticed to Dr. Chandler at Rotherhithe near the East London docks, and he never forgot the mixture of poverty and ignorance which he saw there. He was too young to be admitted to the University of London so studied in the Library of the College of Surgeons whenever he could. [It is impossible to pay sufficient tribute to this Library, the glory of a great profession and the sanctuary of the serious student of medicine for generations. Its rebuilding after direct bomb hits in World War II has been a godsend to a new generation of students.]

Through Sydenham College Huxley was able to prepare for the matriculation examinations of the University of London, in which he won the Medal of the Apothecaries Society for his paper in Botany. With his brother, J. E. Huxley, he entered Charing Cross Hospital Medical College in October, 1842.

We have in Huxley's own words the essence of his student discovery: "The only instruction from which I obtained the proper effect of education was that which I received from Mr. Wharton Jones, who was the lecturer on physiology. . . . The extent and precision of his knowledge impressed me greatly, and the severe exactness of his method of lecturing was quite to my taste. I do not know that I have ever felt so much respect for a teacher before or since. . . . It was he who suggested the publication of my first scientific paper—a very little one—in the *Medical Gazette* of 1845, and most kindly corrected the literary faults which abounded in it."

Possibly Huxley's attendance at post mortem examinations had sharpened his interest in microscopic structures. At all events he spent so much time over the microscope that his classmates, seeing him from the courtyard outside, dubbed him "The Sign of the Head and the Microscope."

Thus at the age of nineteen Huxley wrote his first paper "On a hitherto undescribed structure in the human hair sheath," still known as "Huxley's layer." He continued his brilliant record by winning the prize in chemistry, and at graduation in 1845 won the gold medal for anatomy and physiology.

He immediately joined the Naval Medical Service and under the kindly eye of Sir John Richardson, the explorer and naturalist, was posted as Assistant Surgeon to H. M. S. Rattlesnake about to set off for Australia. Delays there were as noted in his diary: "December 10, 1846. In Plymouth Sound. Thank God! Fitting out is at last over. We have no more caprices to fear but those of the wind—a small matter after having been exposed to those of the Admiralty."

For all his success at University he was commendably cautious as he wrote: "I must keep two points in view, 1st that I *am* simply a student; 2nd from the peculiar circumstances in which I am placed, care and caution in observation may help me to *become* a teacher with regard to particular points."

In the period of more than seven months which it required to reach Australia Huxley had time to ruminate further: "Naturalizing for systematic purposes is not *à mon gré*. My memory is not sufficiently selective of these facts to give me any hope of attaining profound systematic knowledge—and furthermore all the naming and determining of place is far better done by those who sit in museums at home. . . . But what I *can* do and they *cannot* and where therefore the chief value of my position is: I can observe 1. the 'habits' of living bodies, 2. their mode of development and generation, 3. their anatomy by dissection of the fresh specimens, 4. their histology by microscopic observation." Obviously he was still Wharton Jones' disciple, now in action. It speaks well, too, of the value of a medical training when a man sets out to observe even the lowest forms of life clinically, in their habitat, and before they reach a museum.

Huxley's years with the Rattlesnake were varied and interesting. Ashore he was observant too, and noted that even in 1847 he witnessed an operation in Hobart, Tasmania, done under ether anaesthesia, which had been introduced less than a year previously by a Boston medical student.

Huxley became engaged in Sydney to Henrietta Heathorn and they were married in England eight years later; they lived to raise eight children.

On his return with H. M.S. Rattlesnake to England in 1850 Huxley tried to find a publisher for his scientific papers. The Admiralty could not be interested. Huxley therefore resigned his commission and appealed to the Royal Society which responded nobly, thanks to a grant from H. M. Government! Such Peter versus Paul methods of financing research are still standard practice today.

At the age of 25 Huxley was made Fellow of the Royal Society and a year later was awarded its gold medal and elevated to its Council! Despite this the poor man was turned down for posts he sought at the Universities of Toronto, Cork, Aberdeen and at King's College, London. His mother died, his father took ill and Huxley was on the point of settling in Australia as a general practitioner when The School of Mines in London appointed him lecturer in paleontology.

With this appointment began forty years of ceaseless work, turning out scientific papers, sitting on Royal Commissions, on the London School Authority, and as a Governor of Eton. The publication of Darwin's *Origin of Species* in 1859 was Huxley's great opportunity to become a teacher to a whole generation. His speeches and writings soon attracted universal attention. His subjects were not confined to evolution but ranged over the whole field of knowledge. He was a pioneer in adult education, and always the poor man's friend. Injustice, prejudice and privilege he excoriated. His lay sermons in the modern vernacular may be said to have "comforted the afflicted and afflicted the comfortable." Amidst all his crusading he found time to establish in 1871 the first true "laboratory of biology." He founded two scientific journals which may be considered the forerunners of the modern *Nature*. He was best known in America for his appearance at the opening of the Johns Hopkins University where he spoke "On University Education."

From the age of 15 Huxley felt keenly the injustice of a state-supported church. In 1860 Oxford heard even stronger views when he debated the subject of evolution with Bishop Samuel Wilberforce. The Bishop asked if it was through his grandfather or his grandmother that Huxley claimed descent from a monkey. Huxley's classic reply was this: "I asserted—and I

THE CHIEF

1873

His brow spreads large and placid, and his eye
Is deep and bright, with steady looks that still.
Soft lines of tranquil thought his face fulfil—
His face at once benign and proud and shy.
If envy scout, if ignorance deny,
His thoughtless patience, his unyielding will,
Beautiful gentleness and splendid skill,
Innumerable gratitudes reply.
His wise rare smile is sweet with certainties,
And seems in all his patients to compel
Such love and faith as failure cannot quell.
We hold him for another Herakles,
Battling with customs, prejudice, disease,
As once the son of Zeus with Death and Hell.

W. E. HENLEY (1849-1903).

repeat—that a man has no reason to be ashamed of having an ape for his grandfather. If there were an ancestor whom I should feel shame in recalling it would rather be a man—a man of restless and versatile intellect—who, not content with equivocal success in his own sphere of activity, plunges into scientific questions with which he has no real acquaintance, only to obscure them by aimless rhetoric, and distract the attention of his hearers from the real point at issue by eloquent digressions and skilled appeals to religious prejudice."

So we leave Huxley at the end of his threescore years and ten. Without his talents Darwin's theory would never have been so widely spread, and education in Britain would have been the poorer. From a medical student who had one superb teacher who helped him with the faltering report of his little discovery, Huxley became one of the greatest teachers of the last century, a contributor and editor of the top rank, and a scientist-statesman with few equals.

Joseph Lister (1827-1912) *

We have seen the determinative influence of Wharton Jones on the student life of Thomas Huxley in 1845. In 1852 we find this great teacher of physiology influencing another student investigator, Joseph Lister, at University College, London. Having come to the medical school with a B.A. degree, and being skilled in microscopy through association with his father's researches on achromatic lenses, Lister was attracted to the physiological laboratory of Professor William Sharpey. Wharton Jones was still closely associated with physiology though immersed in clinical work.

Lister's excellent microscopy was the key with which he unlocked the secrets of the muscle of the iris, and that of the skin, in two undergraduate studies. He wrote in his first paper, "Observations on the contractile tissue of the iris": "Our knowledge of the cause of the movements of the iris was, till within the last few

* Lister's father-in-law, James Syme (1799-1870), Professor of Clinical Surgery at Edinburgh (1833-1869), at the age of seventeen discovered that naphtha would dissolve crude rubber, thus opening the way to rubberized clothing—still known as "Macintoshes"—after Charles Macintosh who patented the process.

years, in a very unsatisfactory condition. . . . An operation for artificial pupil, by excision, performed by Mr. Wharton Jones at University College Hospital, on the eleventh of August of the present year (1852), placed in my possession a perfectly fresh portion of a human iris. . . . I proceeded to avail myself of this somewhat rare opportunity of investigating the muscular tissue of the human iris. On placing under the microscope, four hours after the operation, portions of the tissue carefully teased out in water with needles, I found that some of the muscular fibre-cells had become isolated, and presented very characteristic appearances."

This paper was published in the first volume of the *Quarterly Journal of Microscopic Science* in 1853, as was his second paper, "Observations on the muscular tissue of the skin." This paper showed the minute muscles which elevate the hairs on the skin surface during fright or other suitable stimulation.

It may seem to some that Lister's excursion into muscle structure and function had no connection with his later work. The common denominator was his superb microscopy. If ever Pasteur's dictum "Fortune favors the prepared mind" was applicable it was to Lister. He saw everything he investigated in physiological terms. In this he was ahead of his time, though in time with his teachers, Sharpey, Wharton Jones and Robert Liston the surgeon. Undoubtedly his boyhood interest in botany had stimulated the inquisitive part of his nature.

Thus an outbreak of "hospital gangrene" in London caused Lister to ask its basic causes. At Edinburgh, where he became an extramural lecturer in surgery in 1853, Lister began his researches on coagulation of the blood and inflammation in the web of the frog's foot.

Lister had learned and practised the essentials of physiological observation as an undergraduate and these he now brought to his clinical problems of what he called "sepsis" and "putrefaction" in wounds. He reasoned from Pasteur's experiments on putrefaction in organic matter that micro-organisms could be at the root of putrefaction in his patients' tissues.

It was thus in May 1866, in Glasgow, that he first treated suppurating wounds with "crude German creosote." Soon after this carbolic acid was isolated and came to be used. Lest we think

Lister was satisfied with this fierce chemical treatment of human tissues we should read Sir Howard Florey's "Lister Oration" to the Canadian Medical Association in Vancouver in 1954. He reproduces Lister's notes of one hundred years ago, from which it is clear that he was in search of an antibiotic to curb infection!

Lister's pre-eminence as a surgeon has tended to obscure the fundamental apprenticeship which he served in physiology. He always urged upon his students his view that it is "by collateral knowledge that healing is most frequently advanced."

Santiago Ramón y Cajal (1852-1934)

No story of student contributions to anatomy would be complete without a reference to the colorful Spaniard, Don Santiago Ramón y Cajal. His rise from the lowliest teaching post to the Nobel Prize in medicine is a romance in itself. What he did for science in Spain—now lost, alas, since the Civil War—is a record of one man against all the elements—poverty, ignorance and prejudice.

Cajal, to use his mother's name, was born in the villa of Petilla de Aragon, the son of a "barber surgeon second class." The most mischievous boy for miles around, Santiago became a legendary figure when he hollowed out a tree trunk and, making an unusually successful cannon of it, blew down the wall of a grandee's palace. Time spent in jail failed to temper his high spirits, but his father's hunting activities were soon shared with him. Together they tramped the hills in search of game, and eventually Santiago developed his flair for drawing and sketching. By judicious visits to cemeteries he built up a fine collection of human bones which he drew to perfection. By the age of 18 he had completed a most creditable atlas of osteology. It was never published, since in Spain foreign medical volumes were the rule. However, the sheets from the atlas, once displayed at the Instituto Cajal in Madrid, were both beautiful and faithful. Like a lot of other things scientific in Spain they are missing today.

By dint of great sacrifice Santiago and his brother graduated with the degree Bachelor of Medicine from the University of Zaragoza. Santiago became lecturer in microscopic anatomy in Valencia and his brother went off to South America where for

30 years he was private secretary to some king of the Pampas, returning to Zaragoza to become Professor of Gynecology!

In Valencia Cajal wrote a set of notes for his students in histology, as Osler did in Montreal at about the same time, and came to the conclusion that there was little to write about on the microscopic structure of the nervous system. The knowledge of this important part of the body was hidden in an impossible thicket of ignorance and speculation. All that our other student contributors Remak and Helmholtz could do with the staining methods at hand was not enough to make much difference.

At this stage Cajal went to Madrid to take his higher degree of Doctor of Medicine. He saw there for the first time the capillary circulation in the web of the frog's foot—the preparation which was to serve Lister so well. He found a psychiatrist in Madrid named Simarro, who had beautiful silver-stained preparations of nervous tissue. Some he had stained by his own method, and some after the method of Camillo Golgi, the Italian anatomist of Pavia.

On Cajal's return to Valencia he began to stain the nervous system of insects and mice. He had so little money that he had to put many sections on one microscope slide. What he saw excited him. He wrote his first paper and sent it to *The Catholic Daily* in Zaragoza. He sent reprints of it to the crowned heads of Europe but received no glowing acknowledgements. Undeterred he stained more minute structures and wrote more papers. He was made Professor at Barcelona and eventually at Madrid. Here the voice of scorn came repeatedly to his ears—who did this Cajal think he was, writing papers for journals beyond the Pyrenees?

Cajal had come out of his laboratory in 1885 to give help in a serious cholera epidemic which swept Spain—and for this help he was given a beautiful microscope by the people of Zaragoza. In the same epidemic there appeared on an English team of researchers sent out by St. Thomas' Hospital, London, a man who was to make Cajal's name famous. He was Charles Sherrington, also destined to receive the Nobel Prize in medicine—and in the same branch of medicine, the study of the nervous system. They did not meet in Spain, but Sherrington learned enough Spanish to read Cajal's papers which came to him later when he was Secretary of the Royal Society in London.

Sherrington, whose research on the physiology of the nervous system began while he was a student, found in Cajal's little papers the structural facts which his physiological experiments made him surmise. Before long he had Cajal invited to London to give the Croonian Lectures at the Royal Society. From that day Cajal never looked back, and the sceptics in Spain were silenced. Sherrington had some fine lantern slides made of Cajal's microscopic specimens, but Cajal refused to show them. He wanted his audience to look into real microscopes to see real structures, and his strategy worked. There was nothing aloof about the reception of his work in Britain. Cambridge accorded him an honorary degree, and Oxford Colleges dipped into their archives to find that they had ancient connections with Spanish Universities, such as Salamanca.

This was all very well, but Cajal's curiosity overcame him, and at times when he should have been getting an honor he would be found in a botanical garden. He arose early and every morning took up his place before eight o'clock at one of the bridges over the Thames, to watch the millions come to work in the city.

Cajal became recognized abroad, and finally in Spain. He was made a life Senator and a great Instituto Cajal was built to honor him. He preferred to work at home, however, writing and editing, and, like a picador, sharpening his lances for the endless polemics which he carried on with opponents of his "neurone theory." His speech on receiving the Nobel Prize in 1906—a prize shared with his caustic opponent Golgi—was a masterpiece of scientific prose. Golgi's was, unhappily, a bitter denunciation of his rival!

Cajal did for the finer anatomy of the nervous system what Vesalius did for gross anatomy. He described what was there to be seen, rather than what authorities decreed to be there. Both began as student contributors, dependent upon the dry bones of gallows and cemeteries. Both left us in their debt.

Frederick Augustus Dixey (1855-1935)

Wherever butterflies are studied the name of Dixey is known. Until recently, however, his name has been forgotten in the field of anatomy relating to the development of bone. Dixey has been truly referred to as a "pioneer of osteogeny."

Frederick Dixey was born at No. 3 New Bond Street, London, in 1855. His grandfather was optician to Queen Victoria and his father followed the same profession. Frederick received his early training at Highgate School under Dr. Dyne, and proceeded to Wadham College, Oxford, with a scholarship in classics. He took his B.A. degree in 1878 and went on to University College, London. There he demonstrated in physiology for Sir Edward Sharpey-Schafer, who later married his sister. Dixey qualified for his B.M. and B.Ch. degrees at Oxford in 1884 and a year later was made Wills Medical Fellow of Wadham College. In 1891 he was awarded his M.D. by Oxford, and thereafter filled a succession of posts in his College as Science Tutor, Bursar and Sub-Warden, being elected an Emeritus Fellow in 1927.

His fame as an entomologist was such that he was elected President of the Entomological Society of London in 1909, and was made a Fellow of the Royal Society in 1910. His scientific interests were broad. He wrote on vital statistics, the epidemiology of influenza and the natural history of diphtheria. He was a confirmed Darwinian. In his College he was noted for his interest in music and in rowing. For thirty-nine years he was a Governor of the Warneford Hospital in Oxford, and a well known churchman.

Our interest lies in his student researches into the development of the bones of the fingers and toes. He was the first to demonstrate that although the shaft of bone making up the terminal phalanx of a digit is laid down in cartilage, its tip and "ungual tuberosity" are laid down in membrane. The plate on p. 39 shows the thimble-like cap of membrane bone developing at the terminal part of the digit, as distinct from the cartilagenous bone of the proximal part of the phalanx.

Because Dixey's account has been forgotten, and is often catalogued under Sir Edward Sharpey-Schafer's name because he it was who communicated the student's paper to the Royal Society in 1879, the main conclusions of his paper (and its amplification in 1880) are given:

"In the ungual phalanx it (the ossification in cartilage) is first seen to arise in the tip or distal extremity of the cartilage, from which it spreads gradually backwards towards the base of the phalanx. Similarly, the subperiosteal deposit of membrane bone in all other cases begins as a thin and narrow ring surrounding the shaft and placed midway between the two extremities, that is to say, in direct relation with the spot where the cartilage first begins to calcify; in the ungual phalanx, however, still preserving its relation with the point of commencing calcification in the cartilage, the deposit of subperiosteal bone first appears as a thin layer closely applied to the tip of the cartilage and fitting over it like a cap. . . . The deposition of new bone along the outer surface of this cap or thimble may take place relatively much more quickly at the summit than at the sides, so that an expansion is formed, which may be of considerable size and which no doubt bears a relation to the conformation of the future nail, hoof or claw. The next stage in the development of the bone is marked by the eruption of the subperiosteal tissue with blood vessels and osteoblasts into the shaft at or near the point where the cartilage first began to calcify. This point in all other cases will be found about the middle of the shaft, but in the ungual phalanx, as has been seen, at the tip."

Dixey was knocked down by a motor car in 1935, as he was crossing Park Lane on his way to a meeting of the Entomological Society, and died on January 16th in St. George's Hospital. As his son said, "he died with his mind full of the work he hoped to do."

In an obituary notice *The Lancet* remarked: "Both in the subjects which he chose for investigation and in the manner of their treatment we can see the value of his previous work in medical fields." It may be said that Frederick Dixey carried on the Christopher Wren tradition at Wadham College of the cultivation of diversity of scientific interests.

"Conrad Gesner, who kept open house . . . for all learned men who came into his neighborhood . . . was not only the best naturalist among the scholars of his day, but of all men of that century he was the pattern man of letters. He was faultless in private life, assiduous in study, diligent in maintaining correspondence and goodwill with learned men in all countries, hospitable—though his means were small—to every scholar who came into Zurich. Prompt to serve all, he was an editor of other men's volumes, a writer of prefaces for his friends, a suggestor to young writers of books on which they might engage themselves and a great helper to them in the progress of their work. But still, while finding time for services to other men, he could produce as much out of his own study as though he had no part in the life beyond its walls."

HENRY MORLEY, 1854.

→

PLATE 2

(a) Joseph Lister's student drawing of the fine muscles of the skin which cause the hairs to stand erect. From the *Quarterly Journal of Microscopical Science*, *1*:262-268, 1853. Courtesy of the Clarendon Press, Oxford.

(b) T. H. Huxley at the age of twenty-one. From: Huxley, Leonard: *Life and Letters of T. H. Huxley*, New York, 1903. Courtesy of Macmillan and Co. Ltd.

(c) Ward's undergraduate sketch of his "triangle" in the neck of the femur. From: Dobson, Jessie: Pioneers of Osteogeny, *Journal of Bone and Joint Surgery*, *31B*:596-599, 1949. Courtesy of the Editor.

(d) F. A. Dixey's student drawing of the developing terminal phalanx in the human. From: Dobson, Jessie: Pioneers of Osteogeny, *Journal of Bone and Joint Surgery*, *33B*: 275-277, 1951. Courtesy of the Editor, and of the Royal Society, London.

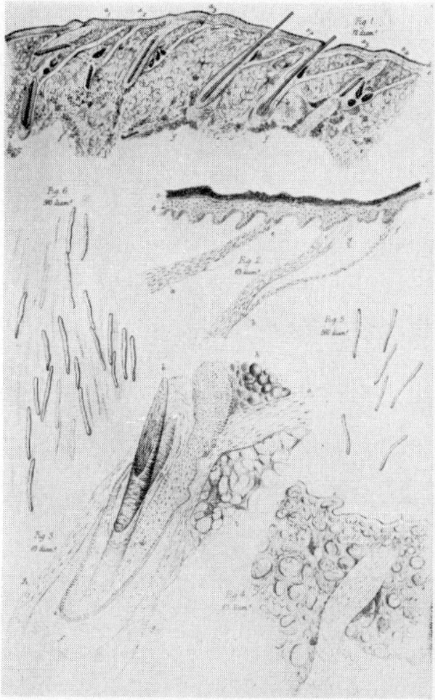

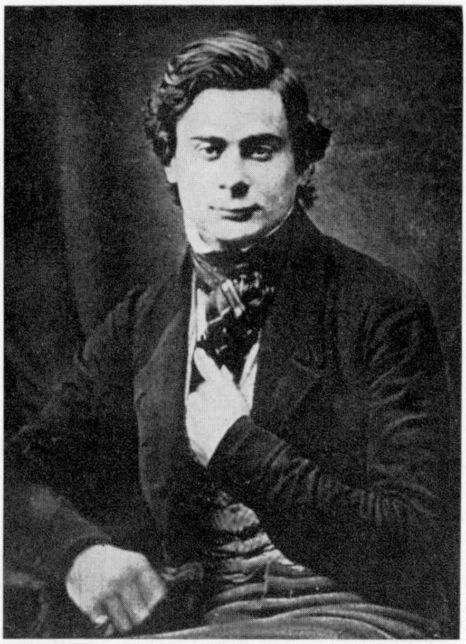

which *a* is the principal support, and *b* a cross piece tying *a* to the wall or column which sustains the whole. It is evident that the piece *a* contributes by its *rigidity*, and the piece *b* by its *tenacity*, to the support of the weight;

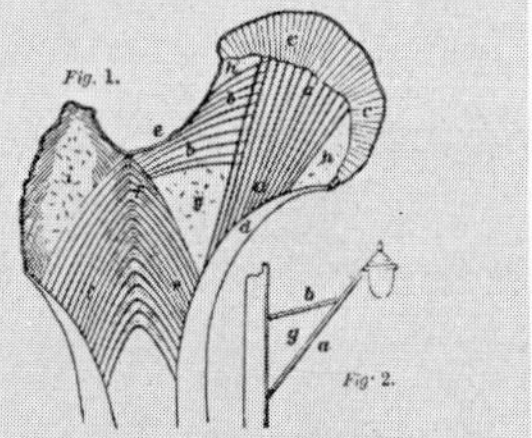

in other words, that the weight tends to *bend* the former, and to *stretch* the latter. Referring to Fig. 1 (in which the direction of the principal fibres is shown with fictitious

FIGS. 1 and 2
Reproduced from page 370 of "Human Osteology" by Oldfield Ward.

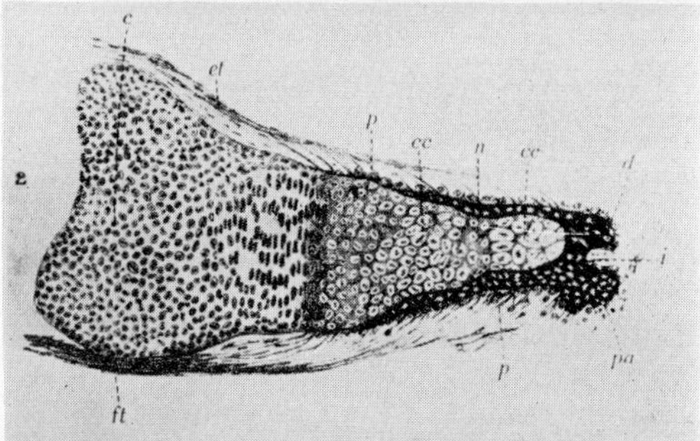

FIG. 1
Sagittal section through the terminal phalanx of the right little finger of a four-month human embryo. (Reproduced here, by permission, from the *Proceedings* of the Royal Society 1880, 1.)

←

Chapter III

Bibliography

PROGRESS IN MEDICINE has depended more upon the written word than it has in any other branch of science. The scholars who, because of their own trials in self-education were determined to simplify the use of the world's literature, form an interesting group of men. Each was a profound scholar of Nature as well as an innovator in the field of bibliography. They enter into our orbit here because they began their work as bibliographers while undergraduate students—doubtless while the iron was hot and when their own personal struggle to codify knowledge was their daily occupation.

Conrad Gesner (1516-1565) is the first of these great men. Osler said that he did not know if Gesner should be placed in his Bibliotheca Prima, where the greatest scientific contributors were arrayed, but added, "But I love him so much I must put him there. Besides he is the father of bibliography." Gesner, the son of a poor furrier in Zurich, graduated in medicine in Basel in 1541 after enduring many privations. Gesner's education was undertaken by his great-uncle, Hans Frick, a man with an interest in botany which was soon communicated to his student. In addition, a dedicated teacher by the name of J. J. Amman took this remarkable lad into his own home and tutored him for three years in Latin and Greek.

Gesner's father was killed as he fought beside Zwingli in the War of the Protestant Reformation, so that Conrad, aged 15, had again to seek help, which he found in the home of the Strasbourg scholar, Wolfgang Capito, where he learned Hebrew. At the age of 16, with a small bursary from Zurich, he set off for France and unfortunately encountered nothing but closed minds at the University of Paris. Returning to Switzerland to teach classics, Gesner began to prepare for his study of medicine. In time, he went to Montpellier, and in 1541 completed his medical doctorate in Basel. It was in the course of his undergraduate studies that he became convinced, as Billings was to be convinced also—300 years later—of the need for the orderly recording and description of all books which would assist scholars in pursuing knowledge.

He had already begun to gather material for his *Bibliotheca Universalis*, an attempt to list and annotate the titles of all books in Greek, Latin and Hebrew ever published. Only youth can start such projects. Even the erudite Gesner little dreamed that his catalogue would reach twenty volumes. Ironically his volume on medical books (Volume XX) was never completed.

Gesner was at once a great botanist, zoologist and scholar, editing the works of the brilliant Valerius Cordus (see page 3), who, in his teens, revolutionized botany, and first synthesized ether. Gesner's bibliographic methods have long been applied in all fields of knowledge, not merely in the medical.

Gesner died of pleurisy at the age of 49, worn out by twenty years of incessant work—his practice by day and his writing by night on his bibliography, on his Greek dictionary, his volumes of botany, his five volume *Historia Animalium*, and his book of selected readings from contemporary surgeons. He was ennobled in the year before his death. For a man who was dogged by poor health and poor eyesight he set a record for creative activity.

Albrecht von Haller (1708-1777), also a Swiss scholar, was a child prodigy, born in Berne into an aristocratic family. His immense bibliographical papers began with his own compilation of two thousand short biographies from his own pen at 8 years of age, and with the writing of a Greek dictionary with Chaldee

"If we think of the Eighteenth Century merely as an age of incisive thinking of materialism and anthropolatry, an age of conscientious clearness, of polish, of self-conceit, as well as skepticism, then Carlyle is right and Voltaire is its chief exponent and representative. But while the conflict with authority was carried on outwardly by the polemics of Voltaire and the literary industry of the encyclopedists, the predominant features, the essential facts of the movement, were the peremptory spirit of free enquiry, together with laborious research and broad systemization. The results of these efforts were utilized by Voltaire and his associates as sturdy weapons of offense. The best minds were inflamed by an inexhaustable and universal curiosity. It was not sometimes in politics and sometimes in religion, as formerly, but in religion, politics, philosophy, man and society, moral and physical sciences, all, everything, became at once the object of study, doubt, and system. In all this it was Haller who was the High Priest; he not only attended the altar, but developed the ceremonials. He was the paragon and epitome of the period. He lived his religion and exemplified it. Voltaire only preached."

C. B. Reed, 1916.

of Dr. Francesco Cordasco of Long Island University (republished by William F. Kelleher, New York, 1950). Watt opened his "Address to medical students on the best method of prosecuting their studies" thus:

> It is not from having spent a certain number of years at schools of medicine, it is not from having repeatedly paid fees to the most eminent teachers, nor from the charm of degrees, diplomas and other academical honors, that diseases are to be cured. No, it requires real medical skill, and that can only be acquired from diligent and unwearied exertion.
>
> The reading of the student is too often confined to systems and to compilations, which are generally the works of men of no experience, or of men writing under the influence of preconceived opinions. By the first, materials of little value are as readily selected as those of real importance; while, by the last, only such facts are recorded as go to support a particular theory. To obtain correct views in medicine it is necessary to have recourse to original writers, to such as write from actual observation, who have seen and treated the diseases they describe.
>
> Many students, however, are neither possessed of such works or have access to them. To remedy this defect, the present plan of establishing a Library is undertaken and it is hoped that it will meet the approbation of those for whose benefit it is intended.
>
> In my lectures on the Practice of Medicine, after considering the history and treatment of each disease, I give a list of the best authors who have written on that subject, and I now put it in your power to peruse these authors, to examine their facts and opinions, and to draw your own conclusions! The sooner you begin to investigate such topics and decide for yourselves, the sooner will you arrive at a true knowledge of your profession. You are thus enabled to collect a stock of ideas, not the tenets of this author or of that teacher, but the result of your own research and discrimination.

He was clearly not speaking to those to whom James Atkinson, his predecessor, addressed his *Medical Bibliography*—"To all idle medical students in Great Britain."

While all of this is of interest to us, Watt's reputation rests largely upon his monumental *Bibliotheca Britannica*. This was developed gradually by the addition, to the medical titles, of works in law, divinity, and other subjects. At the age of forty-three, Watt had a premonition of his early death and wrote that, "He saw himself verging towards the afternoon of life in an impaired state of health." Accordingly he retired to Campvale and there worked until his death two years later on his *Bibliotheca Britannica* or a "General Index to the Literature of Great Britain and Ireland Ancient and Modern, including such foreign works as have been translated into English or printed in the British Dominions, as also a copious selection of the writings of the most distinguished authors of all ages and nations." From his sick-bed he supervised the work of his two literary sons and just before his death a few sheets of this first section came to his sick bed from the printers. Four hundred subscribers are listed as having contributed to the support of the publication. The sons died of tuberculosis and Watt's widow received nothing from the publisher, who failed. The 50,000 titles dealt with were found on slips of paper in the two sacks already mentioned as being among the possessions of Watt's penniless and insane daughter. Today they fill fifteen volumes on authors and fifty-four volumes on subjects in the Paisley Free Library. Thus Watt's undergraduate dream of someday preparing a great bibliography of published works in English, was realized.

John Shaw Billings (1838-1913)

"There is no better float through posterity than to be the author of a good bibliography."

—Osler

Some will wonder at the inclusion of John Shaw Billings in a work on student discoverers. Billings, as an undergraduate, made a discovery which influenced the lives of more potential medical discoverers than any other single development in medical literature.

He was born in Cotton Township in Switzerland County, Indiana, on April 12, 1838. His father ran a country cross-roads store at Allensville. The family moved to Rhode Island to farm but later returned to Indiana. They were originally descended from John Howland who came to America on the Mayflower, and through every vicissitude and tribulation in the West maintained one thing which is central to our theme—the New Englanders' love of literature.

At an early age John Shaw Billings became saturated with the printed word, and by the age of eight he had read the Bible through completely. At the age of ten he embarked on the study of Latin, with a grammar, a copy of Caesar and a dictionary. Fortunately he found a ready and sympathetic tutor in the local cleric. He taught himself Greek and geometry and on the strength of these entered Miami University at Oxford, Ohio, at the age of fourteen!

Having already learned to study by himself, he was able to carry his college work with ease. Thus he found time to browse in the University's eight thousand volume library. This collection was remarkable chiefly for the fact that it could only be consulted on Saturday mornings, at which time each student could borrow two books!

While not "exophthalmic with bibliomania" as Harvey Cushing used to say of some of his book-collecting colleagues, Billings definitely became an addict in his early years—later, of course, he was characterized by Dr. Oliver Wendell Holmes as "a bibliophile of such eminence" that he regarded him "as a positive danger to the owner of a library if he is ever let loose in it alone."

Living on seventy-five cents a week—mostly on milk and eggs according to Weir Mitchell—Billings had no money for entertainment. He was of a practical turn of mind, however, and quickly found a method of climbing into the university library on six days of the week, so that he had, in effect, a private library of eight thousand volumes. He sampled a wide variety of them, and the broad knowledge gained there enabled him to tutor other students, as a means of supporting himself.

In 1857 Billings graduated near the top of his class and became a "lecturer" with a touring magic lantern show. By 1858 he had earned enough money to enable him to enter the Medical College of Ohio, founded by Daniel Drake (now the University of Cincinnati).* He graduated in 1860 after a concentrated course,

* The pioneer educator and physician of "the West," Daniel Drake, published his famous geographical study of disease, "Climate and Diseases of Cincinnati," in 1810, five years before he took his M.D. degree at Philadelphia. Though he began his medical apprenticeship at age 15 his formal training at Philadelphia was often interrupted by financial crises. Born in poverty in New Jersey he nevertheless rose to the top of America's profession, founded two medical schools, and wrote the finest papers on medical education of the early nineteenth century.

made doubly so by his simultaneous employment as caretaker of the dissecting rooms. In addition, he "lived in" at one of the hospitals.

Billings' undergraduate "discovery" was made in the performance of "that melancholy duty" of writing a graduation thesis, in 1860. What he found greatly influenced his life, as he relates it:

"This has happened in this wise: In the thesis just referred to, it was desirable to give the statistics of the results obtained from certain surgical operations as applied in the treatment of epilepsy. To find these data in their original and authentic form required the consulting of many books, and to get at these books I not only ransacked all the libraries, public and private, to which I could get access in Cincinnati, but for those volumes not found here (and these were the greater proportion), search was made in Philadelphia, New York and elsewhere, to ascertain if they were in any accessible libraries in this country.

"After about six months of this sort of work, and correspondence, I became convinced of three things. The first was, that it involves a vast amount of time and labor to search through a thousand volumes of medical books and journals for items on a particular subject, and that the indexes of such books and journals cannot always be relied on as a guide to their contents. The second is, that there are in existence somewhere, over one hundred thousand volumes of such medical books and journals, not counting pamphlets and reprints. And the third was, that while there was nowhere in the world a library which contained all medical literature, there was not in the United States any fairly good medical library, one in which a student might hope to find a large part of the literature relating to any medical subject, and that if one wished to do good bibliographical work to verify the references given by European medical writers, or to make reasonably sure that one had before him all that had been seen or done by previous observers or experimenters on a given subject, he must go to Europe and visit, not merely one, but several of the great capital cities in order to accomplish his desire.

"It was this experience which led me, when a favourable

opportunity offered at the close of the war (1865) to try to establish, for the use of American physicians, a fairly complete medical library, and in connection with this to prepare a comprehensive catalogue and index which should spare medical teachers and writers the drudgery of consulting ten thousand or more different texts, or of turning over the leaves of as many volumes to find the dozen or so references of which they might be in search."

Following graduation, Billings acted as Demonstrator in Anatomy at his *alma mater* and was about to enter surgical practice when the Civil War supervened. Passing at the top of a list of applicants he was appointed First Lieutenant and Assistant Surgeon in April, 1862, and sent to Cliffburne General Hospital, Washington, D.C. This institution he found to be "in an extremely filthy and dilapidated condition—no drainage whatever, no sinks, no water within half a mile." How it had served formerly as the barracks of the Fifth United States Cavalry is hard to imagine. However, Billings plunged in, and his career as designer and builder of hospitals began!

Billings' Army career was intensely interesting and varied. In 1863 he was sent to work under Surgeon General of the Army of the Potomac, Jonathan Letterman. In the Battle of Chancellorsville he had the experience "of handling wounded without an ambulance corps, and getting them off when the troops were falling back. . . . We lost altogether between ten and fifteen thousand men." At the Battle of Gettysburg he operated on casualties for seven days continuously—yet found time to keep up his case notes and statistics on the number of gunshot wounds, cases of tetanus and secondary haemorrhages.

These details of Billings' already colourful career are cited as proof of the man's sheer ability and physical endurance. In 1862, with his successful excision of the ankle joint, he was the forerunner of Lister—another student discoverer—whose oft-quoted case of excision of the wrist was to be published in 1865.

In August of 1864 Billings' field service came to an end, and on the last day of the year he was assigned to the Surgeon General's office in the War Department at Washington. There he was to spend thirty-one productive years, leaving as his memorial, the great Surgeon General's Library and its invaluable *Index Catalogue*.

Billings' great opportunity to follow up his student "discovery" came in 1868, when Surgeon General Barnes—to his eternal credit—gave him a sum of eighty thousand dollars, remaining unspent in Civil War Hospital funds, to establish a medical library worthy of the name. At the time of Billings' arrival in the Surgeon General's office, the library comprised two thousand two hundred fifty-three volumes, indexed in a thirty-one page catalogue. By 1872, the catalogue was four hundred fifty-four pages in length. By the time Billings retired from the Army (1895) the first series of sixteen volumes of the *Index Catalogue* was completed and the next series was about to commence.

Billings achieved his ambition because he knew how to state his case clearly—something he may have learned in his magic-lantern show days—something which he certainly developed in his Civil War service. He was able to establish the *Index Medicus* in 1879 and to get an appropriation from Congress in 1880 to start printing his *Index Catalogue*. Hume has given a most scholarly account of Billings' development of this unique bibliographic enterprise, and gives us some indication of his satisfaction as it developed. "Billings once said that a librarian is in one respect only a sort of hod carrier, who brings together the bricks made by one set of men in order that another set of men may build therewith—but he is apt to take quite as much pride and satisfaction in the resulting structure, provided it be a good one, as if he built it himself."

An undergraduate who aspired to a "private library" of eight thousand volumes, and who recognized too that a real medical bibliographical service was needed in the world, was unlikely to be backward in producing arguments for his "brain child." He simply told the incredulous that "Books are properly compared to tools of which the index is the handle." He bluntly told Congress that the cost of printing his *Index Catalogue* would compare with the cost of an "expedition to the North Pole, five miles of subsidized railroad, one company of cavalry, or a small post office building." In terms of the cost of modern military aircraft, Billings today would undoubtedly have some astronomical but sound demands to make of Congress!

The Washington setting of the Surgeon General's Library and the Army Medical Museum, both of which Billings directed gave additional scope to his broad range of interests. He helped reorganize the Marine Hospitals, and also reported on Army Military Posts. He called the U.S. Army "the best fed and the worst housed army in the world." He advised the Government on matters of vital statistics. In 1880 he suggested that the data compiled from the census "might be recorded on a single card or slip by punching small holes in it, and that these cards might then be sorted and counted by mechanical means according to any selected group of these perforations." It is little wonder that his advice was sought on a multitude of matters.

Thus it was that in 1876 the trustees of Johns Hopkins' Fund asked Billings to become their medical adviser. He entered the competition set up for plans for the Johns Hopkins Hospital, and his were accepted. The debt of Johns Hopkins University to Billings is great indeed. For many years he lectured there on Hygiene, and later on the History of Medicine. The colourful Tom Cullen took a train car full of students to the Surgeon General's Library annually to see Billings and his monumental collection.

Billings found time to act as Chairman of the Board of Trustees of the Carnegie Institution of Washington. The Corporation of the projected Peter Bent Brigham Hospital in Boston asked him to draw up suitable plans for another great teaching hospital, which was completed in the year of Billings' death.

In 1895, on retiring from the Army,* Billings became Professor of Hygiene and Director of the Laboratory of Hygiene at the University of Pennsylvania in Philadelphia. He was induced to leave this post to go to New York to build what is again a monument to his wisdom and ability—the New York Public Library. By welding together the Astor Library—a great reference collection—and the Lenox Library, with the help of the

* Billings chose as his successor the brilliant yellow fever researcher Walter Reed, who tragically died, one week after taking over the Librarianship, of a ruptured appendix.

Tilden Trust, Billings created the basis for the modern library services of New York City. The enabling legislation was passed in 1897, the cornerstone laid in 1902 and the great edifice opened in 1911. Billings' imprint is everywhere to be found in the building itself and in the provisions for the use of the books. One important development was the offer to Billings by Andrew Carnegie, of five million two hundred thousand dollars with which to build sixty-five libraries in New York!

Many people wondered how Billings found time for all this creative activity. To his friend MacAlister of London he replied: "I will let you into the secret. There is nothing really difficult if you only begin. Some people contemplate a task until it looms so big it seems impossible. But I just begin and it gets done somehow. There would be no coral islands if the first bug sat down and began to wonder how the job was to be done."

No summary of the contribution of John Shaw Billings to medicine has been more strikingly put than that by Dr. William Welch, the Doyen of American Medicine, quoted by Hume:

> I have been asked on more than one occasion what have been the really great contributions of this country to medical knowledge. I have given the subject some thought and think that four should be named:
>
> 1. The discovery of anaesthesia.
> 2. The discovery of insect transmission of disease.
> 3. The development of the modern public health laboratory, in all that the term implies.
> 4. The Army Medical Library and its *Index Catalogue*, and this library and its catalogue are the most important of the four.

Chapter IV

Cardio-Vascular System

THE YEARS FROM William Harvey (1578-1657) to Sir Thomas Lewis (1881-1945) are rich in student contributions in the field of the circulation of the blood. In his delightful translation of Harvey's great work *De Motu Cordis*, designed for students, Leake has drawn attention to the fact that William Harvey as a student at Padua assisted his teacher Fabricius of Aquapendente (1537-1619) in experiments. Leake's reference is to observations which Harvey made on chick embryos, about the year 1600 "in the spring season by way of helping out Fabricius" (*De generatione*, exercise 6). Fabricius regarded him as one of his favorite pupils and taught him the virtue of methodical observation. This quality was superimposed upon the background of a basic education at Cambridge at the College of Johannes Caius whom Osler called "the first English student of clinical medicine."

From Fabricius, Harvey learned the method of applying ligatures or cords to blood vessels which he later used to ascertain the direction, volume, and force of the blood's flow. It was from Fabricius, who in 1600 published his *De formatu foetu*, that Harvey also learned the elements of embryology. Commencing his observations in the chick embryo, as Aristotle had done, with "a drop of blood . . . which throbs," Harvey came to consider the flowing blood as more important than the heart itself. He refers repeatedly to the blood's primacy, both in time of development in the embryo and in its functions in the body. From this position his generalization logically followed, of "a continual movement of the blood in a circle . . . caused by the beat of the heart" (1616).

Since, as Michael Foster says, Fabricius "was the first after Aristotle to describe the formation of the chick in the egg," we may assume that Harvey's earliest medical thoughts were laden as much with his teacher's experiments on chick embryos as with those on the valves of the veins. The impression which this early association with an embryologist, interested in vascular systems made upon his apprentice may have been crucial in the discovery which Harvey was to make. Evidence in favor of this view is to be seen in the following passage from *De motu cordis*:

> I have seen the first rudiments of the chick as a little cloud in the hen's egg about the fourth or fifth day of incubation, with the shell removed and the egg placed in clear warm water. In the center of the cloud there was a throbbing point of blood, so trifling that it disappeared on contraction and was lost to sight, while on relaxation it appeared again like a red pin-point. Throbbing between existence and non-existence, now visible, now invisible, it was the beginning of life.

Fabricius had a patient "helper" with his experiments in the year 1600 and the world, sixteen years later, was to learn of the helper's new theory of the circulation of the blood. It is little wonder that Sir Thomas Browne said that he preferred the circulation of the blood to the discovery of America.

Jan Swammerdam (1637-1680)

In the year following Harvey's death a pre-medical student in Holland, Jan Swammerdam (1637-1680), discovered the red corpuscles in the blood of a frog. He wrote: "In the blood I perceived the serum in which floated an immense number of rounded particles, possessing the shape of, as it were, a flat oval, but nevertheless wholly regular. These particles, however, seemed to contain within themselves the humor of other particles. When they were looked at sideways, they resembled transparent rods as it were, and many other figures, according, no doubt, to the different ways in which they were rolled about in the serum of the blood. I remarked besides that the color of the objects was the paler the more highly they were magnified by means of the microscope."

Because of ill health Swammerdam did not enter the medical course at Leyden until 1663. Within a year he had discovered the valves of the lymphatic vessels. In his graduation year he discovered that the lungs of the newborn float if respiration has already taken place. In addition he introduced a method of injecting specimens, using, at first, suet to trace out the blood vessels.

The productivity of this man was unbelievable. He devised micro-scissors and dissecting devices of great intricacy for his work on insects. He studied the irritability of muscles and their nerves after removal from the body. He opposed the theory of spontaneous generation vehemently.

From his injection syringes he was able to make simple plethysmographs for measuring the volume of the heart in systole and diastole.

After a life of intense activity Swammerdam developed "melancholia," and followed the mystic Antoinette Bourignon to Holstein. He died at the age of forty-two. The "Bible of Nature" containing his works was lost until Boerhaave published it in 1737, fifty-seven years after the author's death. It is from Haller's edition of Swammerdam's dissertation on "Respiration" (1667) that our Plate 3(c) is taken. The "*Bible of Nature*" set a new standard for biological illustration.

There have been few scientists who have accomplished as much as Swammerdam in the twenty-two years from his discovery of the red cells of the blood to his death.

Adam Christianus Thebesius (1686-1732)

Adam Christianus Thebesius (1686-1732) studied medicine at Leyden and there conducted anatomical investigations on the coronary vessels of the heart. By injecting a variety of materials into these vessels he was able to demonstrate their connection with small ostia in the endocardium. His findings were published in his graduation thesis at the age of twenty-two, "Disputatio Medica inauguralis de Circulo Sanguinis in Corde" (Leyden, 1708). This

"Thebesian System" was confirmed by Abernethy in 1798, using similar injection procedures.

In passing it may be of interest to note that James Hope (1801-1841) in his graduation thesis at Edinburgh in 1825 wrote on "Aneurism of the Aorta." Six years later he was to produce what is still regarded as a classic, "A treatise on the diseases of the heart and great vessels."

Sir Astley Paston Cooper (1768-1841)

Sir Astley Paston Cooper (1768-1841) was the versatile and gifted son of a Norfolk clergyman. He was the wildest of ten children, and his youthful escapades are said to have interfered with his formal education. Cooper's mother was a descendant of Isaac Newton, and his paternal grandfather was a surgeon. His uncle, William Cooper, was senior surgeon at Guy's Hospital, London, and it was to him that Astley Cooper was apprenticed in 1784, at the age of sixteen.

In London Astley Cooper, with his fellow students Holland and Coleman, lived at the home of Mr. Henry Cline, Surgeon to St. Thomas' Hospital. (Coleman later founded the Veterinary College of London.) In company with Coleman, Cooper made many dissections at Mr. Cline's house, and sought to elucidate the problem of collateral circulation. They tied off the femoral and the brachial arteries in dogs, and with the aid of injection techniques followed out the finest collateral branchings of the vascular tree.

Cooper attended and discussed with his student colleagues the lectures of the famous John Hunter, whose spur was constantly driving another contributor, Edward Jenner, with this injunction: "But why think, why not try the experiment?" For a period of seven months Edinburgh was to know the talented Cooper. So highly was he regarded there by his fellow students that, at the time of his return to London, they offered to elect him to their Presidency if he ever came again to study.

Back in London, Cooper conducted further animal experiments with Coleman, this time on respiration. As a senior student in 1791, he was asked by Mr. Cline to take over a large share of his lecturing in surgery.

Once launched on his surgical career, Cooper developed, in rapid succession, operations for the ligation of the common carotid artery, the external iliac artery and eventually his heroic ligation of the abdominal aorta (1817). He wrote texts on *Hernia*, *Injuries of the Joints*, *Diseases of the Testis*, and the *Thymus Gland*. Students today still speak of Cooper's fascia.

He had broad social sympathies and was an important figure in the life of London. He was a model of industry, and a great teacher. He gave students an unrivalled chance to learn surgery, and was among the first to lecture from patients rather than didactically. He even took students to help him dissect an elephant which died in the menagerie at the Tower of London!

Jean Leonard Marie Poiseuille (1799-1869)

Jean Leonard Marie Poiseuille (1799-1869) was born in Paris and there studied medicine. His graduation dissertation of 1828 "Recherches sur la force du coeur aortique" describes what he called a "haemodynamometer," which was to replace the Rev. Stephen Hales' arterial cannula for the direct measurement of blood pressure.* The introduction of mercury as the registering fluid greatly facilitated clinical and experimental work. This simple instrument was transformed by Karl Ludwig in 1847 into the familiar "kymograph," so omnipresent in the life of medical undergraduates today.

After graduation Poiseuille continued his work in this field, writing in 1830 on "Recherches sur les causes du mouvement du sang dans les veines," and in 1839 on "Mouvement dans les vaisseaux capillaires." In 1840 he began a series of communications to the Academy of Science in Paris which embraced his other great contribution to the science of haemodynamics. His famous biophysical papers enunciated the direct relationship between the speed of currents in a capillary tube and the square of the tube's

* A method for measuring blood pressure in an exposed artery was reported by Rudolf Magnus (1873-1927), while an undergraduate, to the International Congress on Physiology at Bern in 1895. He expanded this work for his graduation thesis at Heidelberg in 1898. He later became one of the world's most eminent physiologists, contributing major discoveries in the field of the pituitary gland, peristalsis in the gut, the maintenance of body posture and the effects of stimulation of the semi-circular canals.

diameter, the pressure and the viscosity of the fluid—still known as Poiseuille's law.

He was a most versatile man, inventing the viscosimeter, and measuring the blood pressure changes occurring with each heart beat, as well as the degree to which arteries dilate with each systole of the heart. He pursued the physics of capillary tubes further. In 1845 he produced a work on the ventilation of ships. He wrote also on respiration, and upon such chemical subjects as the metabolism of glucose and urea. His many contributions to science were recognized by France, and he was fittingly made Officier de la Légion d'Honneur.

Paul-Louis Duroziez (1826-1897)

Another French physician who contributed to cardio-vascular physiology was Paul-Louis Duroziez (1826-1897). While an undergraduate, in 1850, he was awarded the Corvisart Prize for his essay on "Therapeutic properties and physiologic action of digitalis." Like Purkinje, Duroziez was interested in the toxic and delirious states encountered in overdosage with digitalis. Graduating in 1851 he chose as his thesis subject an analysis of the cases admitted during the term 1850-1851 to the service of Professor Bouillaud.

Ten years later Duroziez wrote a paper on the subject with which his name is still closely connected: "Du double souffle intermittent crural, comme signe de l'insuffisance aortique." In 1877 he published an excellent work on "pure mitral stenosis," its sequelae and sex distribution. His *Clinical Treatise on Diseases of the Heart* was widely acclaimed in 1891, and was awarded prizes both by the Academy of Medicine and by the Institute of France.

Duroziez represents the best in general practice in France. He was associated with the clinic at the Charité, but never held a chair nor headed a large hospital service. Nevertheless he is said to have been welcomed universally as a true contributor to medical science. Two years before his death he was made Chevalier de la Légion d'Honneur. His life and works have been chronicled in a student thesis at the University of Paris by Feiga Helfenbein (1922).

Augustus Volney Waller (1816-1870)

The English county of Kent can claim such a student of the heart and blood vessels as William Harvey, just as Shropshire claims clinical observers of the type of Jenner and Withering. To the name of Harvey we should add that of A. V. Waller, whose early brilliant researches on the smallest blood vessels, the capillaries, led him into that field of degeneration in the nervous system known the world over as "Wallerian degeneration."

Though born in Faversham, Kent, Waller studied his medicine in France, a country with which his life came to be closely linked. His researches, curiously enough, revolved about the tongue of the frog, that indestructible friend of medical research which first showed Malpighi the conversion of venous to arterial blood in the capillaries of its lungs—the missing link in Harvey's great generalization, surmised by him but not demonstrated until microscopes were invented. One thinks of Waller in a long line of investigators dependent for the truth upon the frog—Leeuwenhoek; Swammerdam observing the red blood corpuscles; Pfluger, studying the miracle of oxidation in its tissues; Descartes, the physiologist-philosopher, asking it questions; the brothers Weber, working out the slowing of its heart, and our hearts, by stimulating its vagus nerve; Gaskell, finding the nerves which accelerate its heart and our hearts; Johannes Müller and Helmholtz, working out the velocity and direction of nerve impulses in the nervous system; and Joseph Lister, observing inflammation in the web of its foot while he plotted the end of sepsis in surgery.

As a first-year medical student in Paris, Waller watched the coming and going of bood corpuscles through the walls of the microscopic capillary vessels, and he made a beautifully clear and simple drawing of it (Plate 3). This work he published seven years later in *The Philosophical Magazine.* Within three years of this he sent to the Royal Society of London the paper which was to make him famous, on the changes seen in nerves in the frog's tongue when cut off from their mother cells. It was this single fact, more than all others, which eventually caused Ramón y Cajal, Van Gehüchten and Sherrington to grasp the truth now known as "the neurone theory"—that a nerve cell and its fibre processes make up an autonomous unit, which multiplied millions of times gives us our nervous system. Waller, by cutting other nerves in the frog, soon discovered the direction of the nerve impulses to the heart, to the blood vessels of the head, and showed that without an intact retina in the eye there could be no fibres transmitting impulses over the optic nerve to the brain. Thus a medical student with a frog and a microscope became famous.

Maurice Raynaud (1834-1881)

Few physicians have had such "a float through posterity" as Maurice Raynaud was to enjoy. The disease described by him in his Doctor of Medicine thesis we still call "Raynaud's Disease." Raynaud came from a famiy of professors and surgeons. In 1860, two years before he was to write his classic graduation dissertation, "De l'asphyxie locale et de la gangrène symétrique des extrémités," he saw a female patient of twenty-seven years of age in whom all four extremities had spontaneously developed unexplained gangrene. He observed the progress of this patient for a month, and realizing how completely his clinical teachers were at sea as to the origin of this condition, he set out to collect similar cases and to search for a common denominator. He collected twenty already recorded cases and five of his own. In view of the modern criticism that many of his cases would not be considered today as "Raynaud's disease," it may be well to quote from his thesis:

> I am far from attributing the same importance to all of these cases. Some of them are incomplete, some of them are doubtful. . . . I would not be truthful if I did not say that I have certain doubts myself, but there is always a certain interest in the collection, into a single bundle, of certain facts scattered throughout science.

The directness of Raynaud's literary style is a pleasant contrast to the tortured verbiage of our modern times. Under the heading, "Local Syncope of the Most Simple Form," he begins:

"Mme. X., at twenty-six years, has never been ill; but she has been the subject since childhood of an infirmity which makes her an object of curiosity to her acquaintances. Under the influence of very moderate cold, and even at the height of summer, she sees her fingers become ex-sanguine, completely insensible, and of a whitish yellow colour. This phenomenon happens often without reason, lasts a variable time, and terminates by a period of very painful reaction, during which the circulation is re-established little by little and recurs to the normal state. . . . The feet, more impressionable even than the hands, are regularly attacked at meal times and whilst digestion is going on. Menstruation does not appear to have any influence upon the appearance of the phenomenon, but it is a remarkable fact that the complete disappearance of attacks of local syncope has always been noted by this lady as the first index of a commencing pregnancy."

In 1874 Raynaud published a further extensive paper on this disease and, in fact, he maintained his interest in it throughout his all-too-brief life. He died at the age of forty-seven of a long-evident heart disease.

Raynaud was greatly interested in the history of medicine, and in 1862 wrote a delightful book, *La médecine au temps de Molière*, which is still a great source of information on the rigours of French medical education of that period. He pictures the hapless undergraduate being put through a series of inquisitions every two years, to answer the oddest array of questions imaginable, without having had anything but didactic teaching, and thus lacking totally in experience.

The defence of theses by graduating students was a great tribulation to many. The student had to swear that he would obey the laws and the customs designed by the Faculty, that he would attend the mass said for deceased physicians, and finally that he would wage unremitting war upon irregular practitioners. If the senior student survived the examinations, oaths, and gastronomic exercises, he was registered as a physician!

Willem Einthoven (1860-1927)

Every first-year medical student knows something of the anatomy and possibly the social function of the elbow joint, and of the mechanics of its pronation and supination. Few realize that a first-year student in Utrecht in 1879 made an analysis of this mechanism, under the patronage of Koster, the anatomist, and eventually became—not an anatomist—but the father of electrocardiography!

Willem Einthoven was born in Java, the son of a doctor. When Willem was ten years of age his father died, and his mother brought her six children to Utrecht for their education. In 1879 Willem entered the University in Utrecht, and as already described, soon became known as a student of great promise. While still an undergraduate, in 1883, he was given an Assistantship at the Utrecht Eye Hospital and there fell under the spell of Donders and Snellen. Einthoven's graduation thesis was on "Stereoscopic vision through colour differences." While in his final year he was proposed by Donders for the chair of physiology at Leyden, about to be vacated by Heynsius. The chair was offered to him, but, modest undergraduate that he was, he refused it until his associate Carl Koller, of cocaine fame, finally persuaded him to take it and to give up his plan of returning to Java to practise.

A year later Einthoven published a paper "On the law of specific nerve energies," which was to bring immediate recognition to his department at Leyden. He spent the next forty years at Leyden, moving gradually into the physical sciences as applied to clinical problems, and building a great school of able followers.

In order to record the electrical phenomena associated with the heart beat, Einthoven first employed a galvanometer of the d'Arsonval type. He then moved on to a more sensitive instrument of Ader's design used for recording submarine signals by deflections of a wire suspended between the poles of a magnet. By greatly increasing the strength of the magnet, and by decreasing the weight of the suspended wire he arrived at a much more sensitive instrument. The wire's movement was then magnified by an optical projection system and recorded on a camera. By 1909 Einthoven had a recording system one hundred thousand times as sensitive as Ader's original model.

In 1903 Einthoven's classic paper appeared on the galvanometric registering of the human electrocardiogram, with the naming of the P,Q,R,S, and T deflections which we still use. In 1913, with Fahr and de Waart he published the theory of what is still known as "Einthoven's triangle" for deriving the "electrical axis" of the heart.

Einthoven recorded also the electrical impulses passing centrally up the vagus nerve to the brain from the heart. In addition, according to Leonard Hill, he recorded electric variations in the tonus of the sympathetic nervous system. His efforts were all bent to the developing of recording techniques free of inertia and lag. He was able to produce threads of quartz as fine as two millionths of an inch in diameter.

It is a little known fact that as early as 1894, Einthoven and Geluk developed methods for recording heart sounds, and adapted the string galvanometer to register them.

Sir Thomas Lewis has pointed out that the electrical recording of cardiac irregularities brought about an intensive analysis of their mechanism and of the natural history of heart disease. Lewis remarks:

> Einthoven did more than place his wonderful apparatus at the disposal of other workers. He pointed to many of the ways in which it might be employed. Amongst these he called attention particularly to its capacity to portray the electrical events happening in the human heart. Modern electrocardiography, and the analysis of irregular heart action by galvanometric means, may rightly be said to have been inspired by, and in large part founded upon two papers of his published in 1906 and 1908.

Einthoven was a most cultured man, and a great favorite at Leyden—that ancient university which has produced so many brilliant contributors and teachers in medicine. He was awarded the Nobel Prize in 1924 and was made a Foreign Member of the Royal Society of London in 1926. His life was one of teaching and fruitful labor, made happy by the universal acclaim and use of his methods.

John Bruce MacCallum (1876-1906)

A Canadian who contributed to medical knowledge while still an undergraduate medical student is John Bruce MacCallum. Fortunate in his background, MacCallum fulfilled many of his potentialities in his thirty short years of life. When we consider that he published twenty-seven original scientific papers between 1895 and 1906, six of them before his graduation from Johns Hopkins Medical School in 1900, we become aware that we have encountered an unusual personality and intellect. During these same few years, hundreds of letters, many poems and notebooks of memoirs were written which, fortunately, have survived to give us a well-rounded picture of a talented and attractive man and his times.

John Bruce MacCallum will be long remembered for many different reasons. There are still alive people whom he delighted while they were children with his fund of fairy stories—many of them original—and his sketches. Others will recall his love of poetry, music and the theatre, all of which were the themes of many of his most interesting letters and conversations. The enduring monument to his memory will, however, be his contribution to scientific knowledge, those foundations which he laid and upon which other men have based subsequent investigations.

Dr. George A. MacCallum, country doctor and naturalist of note, was the father of a family of four. It would seem that his two sons, John and William, inherited his investigative turn of mind, and perhaps both went on to develop it due to his training and encouragement. All four children, who accompanied their father in turn on his round of professional calls, were taught to enjoy and to observe carefully the birds and plants, large and small, which they passed. From their mother, John and his older sister, at least, inherited a love of music and the latter became an accomplished musician.

Of John B. MacCallum as a boy, we have a picture like that of many of his kind. Scholastically he was outstanding and physically a healthy, sturdy lad. The family did much reading but enjoyed also the pleasures and tasks of the out-of-doors. In 1892 John followed his brother William to the University of Toronto, enrolling in the class of Arts '96. During his first two years there, he revealed in his letters the gloomy moods which were an integral part of his character, although this was apparent to a lesser extent as he matured. The usual period of self-interrogation in youth was, in his case, rather more prolonged than is common. This probably gave rise to his somewhat melancholy poems, some of which were published in Toronto papers.

It was at Toronto in 1895 that John B. MacCallum published his original scientific work, on "Fresh Water Cladocera," which appeared in the *University of Toronto Quarterly*. In this article he instituted his practice of illustrating all his own work.

It is probable that there is always someone in the life of any research-minded student who inspires the first work and whose encouragement and influence are important to its completion. Such a man, in the case of the younger MacCallum brother, was Professor Ramsay Wright, biologist at the University of Toronto. It would be interesting to know just how the spark is kindled, but records of the events or words between teacher and pupil which lead to the discovery of new things are unfortunately only rarely recorded—the case of Edward Jenner and his mentor, John Hunter, being an exception.

During the term 1895-1896 John MacCallum became better adjusted socially and emotionally to his life at the University. He was fond of dancing and the theatre but took little interest in sports. Each moment of his day was used to advantage, although he never then, nor later, seemed to give the impression of being too busy or pressed in spite of the vast amount of work he accomplished. Sometime in this same term his decision was made to attend Johns Hopkins Medical School, where his brother had already gone, and he accordingly registered there in the autumn of 1896.

The next four years record a phenomenal achievement. He published five important original scientific papers, while creditably passing the required examinations in medicine. He published what is still the classical work on the development and architecture of the muscular wall of the heart. It is said that the work for this paper was completed in three weeks in F. P. Mall's laboratory. The same problem had attracted the interest of another medical undergraduate, Gerdy, in Paris, seventy-five years earlier. In addition to his own work he proof-read and indexed *The Nervous System and its Constituent Neurones* by Professor Lewellys F. Barker and maintained a voluminous correspondence with his family and a few friends. Dr. Franklin P. Mall, anatomist and embryologist, and Dr. Simon Flexner who taught pathology, seem to have provided the stimulus for most of his undergraduate research, although undoubtedly the presence of such men as Dr.

William Osler, Dr. Welch, and others, was an additional source of inspiration. Four of John MacCallum's five papers were on the anatomy and pathology of the heart; the remaining one concerned the human sartorious muscle. His illustrations for these papers, particularly those of the heart muscle layers, are beautifully drawn and of great value to his readers. All of these publications were of the utmost significance at a time when histology was not commonly used as a basis for the teaching of anatomy. The knowledge of both structure and function was less complete than it now is.

John Bruce MacCallum, although aware of his talent, remained modest and unassuming. His research was very important to him and, in spite of the apparent ease with which he carried it out, he was under constant strain until each task he set himself was completed. His striving for greater knowledge never ceased and his investigations continued until his death from tuberculosis at the age of thirty. Each one he carried out thoroughly and, consequently, his contribution to basic medical knowledge was very great. As a teacher, both in Denver, Colorado, and at the University of California, he was outstanding and popular, but his scientific research remained always his greatest interest and love.

It is a far cry from Padua to Ontario, and yet the problems faced by Harvey and by MacCallum were similar. Harvey boiled the heart, the better to study its fibrous structure. J. B. MacCallum worked at his problem, and Gerdy's problem, with newer methods, but still with the embryologist's approach. What a pity Harvey did not have the distinguished embryologist Franklin Mall at his elbow! Incidentally, they would have had a great deal in common, for Harvey courted unpopularity by *thinking* about the circulation, and Mall was attacked by some because he used teaching methods designed to make students *think*.

One cannot leave J. B. MacCallum, the undergraduate investigator, without referring to Osler's great affection for him. In the Osler Library at McGill, there is an unpublished manuscript, "Spirit of Death" by MacCallum, given to Osler by Archibald Malloch, MacCallum's talented biographer. The poem concludes:

> "Oh come, be swift and take me while I stand,
> My work still strong beneath a steady hand."

Osler has written beside it:

> One of the most brilliant young men it has ever been my lot to teach. . . . He had a mind of singular acuteness, a clear judgment, and he had caught from Mall some measure of that investigating spirit which has made the anatomical school of the Johns Hopkins University so famous. When the news of his death reached me one morning as I sat at breakfast, I broke down in an irresistible paroxysm of regret, and had to leave the table.

Martin Flack (1882-1931)

Man's translation into the upper atmosphere in self-propelled machines during the last half-century has opened a new chapter of human physiology. Today we assume that fitness to fly must be proven by any person, in civilian or service pursuits, wishing to pilot or navigate an aircraft through the sky. Little do we realize that the tests of such fitness were not always with us—in fact there were none of a scientific nature before World War I. It was soon after the outbreak of that conflict that Martin Flack of the Medical Research Council of Great Britain was charged with the development of standards of fitness to fly. One such test is still known as the Flack test; in it the candidate blows up a column of mercury 40 millimetres high and holds it with all the expiratory force at his command for as long as he can.

Who, then, was Flack? Martin William Flack was born in Kent—that county which has supplied such cardio-vascular student investigators as Harvey and Waller. Martin's father was butcher and grocer in the village of Borden. Martin made his way in the world through scholarships won at school and at the age of nineteen entered Keble College, Oxford, to prepare for a medical career. He was fortunate in the professors under whom he studied—Arthur Thomson and Francis Gotch—and in the friendship of W. H. Jackson, the Radcliffe Librarian, himself a Fellow of Keble.

In the summer of 1903, the village of Borden witnessed the arrival of the great anatomist and teacher, Arthur Keith, at Mann's Place, which delightful spot was to prove a week-end refuge from the unceasing round of London. The butcher's delivery man announced proudly that his master's son, Martin Flack, had recently come down from Oxford and was to commence the clinical part of his training in London. For Arthur Keith this was stimulus enough, and in a twinkling he had Martin Flack enrolled at The London Hospital, and, of course, headed for undergraduate research with Keith.

This partnership was to lead to the discovery of the important "pacemaker" or sino-auricular node of the heart. The work was conducted during the summer of 1906 at Keith's cottage in Kent, where he had assembleld 130 hearts, a microscope, and a microtome for cutting thin sections through small blocks of tissue. One evening on returning from a bicycle ride Arthur Keith found that Flack had come upon a new structure in the right auricle of a mole's heart. It had the microscopic composition of an electrical conducting system but was located far from the then-known auriculo-ventricular conducting fibres. A review of the already prepared slides of other hearts showed this newly found structure to be present consistently. This was indeed a new discovery in the *terra incognita* of the heart. By Christmas of 1906 the student and his professor had their report ready for publication. It appeared in the *Journal of Anatomy* early in 1907 entitled, "The Form and Nature of the Muscular Connections between the Primary Divisions of the Vertebrate Heart."

It is hard to imagine a more important student research than this one, and it bears out the value of close personal collaboration between pupil and professor in an unhurried setting. What was the setting? Sir Arthur Keith's wonderful autobiography recounts the story of their consultations over a game of golf:

> Going to a neighboring chalk ridge on which sheep were grazed (we) laid out a course of nine holes without asking the leave of anyone. With the help of James Braid's manual and our mother wit we set out to learn the great game. We both became infatuated; we would drop our work on the heart to fight out many and many a game. The ridge on which we played was fringed by a belt of wood. That wood swallowed up our supply of balls at an amazing rate.

Flack's reputation as an investigator naturally spread along the corridors of The London Hospital and before long Sir Leonard

Hill snared him for physiological pursuits. Together they investigated many problems in respiration and circulation, in athletes especially, until 1908 when Flack graduated. The following year a Radcliffe Travelling Fellowship enabled him to study with Kronecker and Asher in Switzerland. He returned to work with Hill in London and moved to the Applied Physiology Laboratory of the Medical Research Council with Hill when it was established in 1913.

The First World War saw Flack seconded to the embryo Air Service. From then until his death in 1931 his life was full to overflowing with contributions to aviation medicine. His Milroy Lectures of 1921, delivered before the Royal College of Physicians of London, have preserved, for all to read, the great volume of observations made by trained observers in the First World War. Our present problems of anoxia and hyperventilation and motion sickness were recognized as cardinal problems then. Flack's energy as an investigator and teacher became a legend in the Royal Air Force. Great was the grief of his colleagues in medicine and in aviation when he died in 1931 at the age of fifty of septicemia.

Martin Flack's career illustrates, surely, the value of close informal relations between students with fertile minds and teachers filled with the spirit of scientific adventure. His basic researches and his planning of research establishments in aviation medicine left us all in his debt a short nine years after his death. The pilots who served in the Battle of Britain, the "few" to whom we owed so much, in turn owed much to Martin Flack.

Thomas Lewis (1881-1945)

Finally, Thomas Lewis (1881-1945) comes to mind as an outstanding contributor in the cardio-vascular field, both as an undergraduate and as a graduate student. He was born in Tynant, Cardiff, the son of a wealthy coalmine owner. His preliminary education was pursued at Clifton, near Bristol, but for his preclinical medical training he returned to Wales. Under the guidance of Swale Vincent, Lewis wrote his first paper, at the age of twenty, on the haemolymph glands. His approach and his thoroughness made it a classical paper.

For his clinical work as an undergraduate Lewis went up

to University College Hospital in London. He had failed his London Matriculation examination at the age of sixteen, but he made no mistake about his preparation for the final examinations in medicine; he won the University Medal in 1904 when he graduated! It is of interest and importance to note that he shared lodgings with T. R. Elliott—that unsung genius whose insight, as a very young man, led us to regard the cells of the adrenal medulla as "effector cells" in the sympathetic nervous system through their production of adrenalin.

Lewis served as house surgeon to Victor Horsley, but his apprenticeship was cut short by the fatigue which overtook him, rather prophetically. His other residency was served under Thomas Barlow. Lewis then became caught up in the meshes of research which bound Bayliss, Starling and Cushny together at University College. Lewis began to work on the mechanism of pleural effusion in the laboratory. On the clinical side he received an appointment in 1906 to the staff of the London Chest Hospital. In that year Lewis produced two papers on the alterations in arterial and venous pressures induced by respiratory efforts. His findings differed from those of the outstanding authority Leonard Hill who, typically, thereupon invited Lewis to contribute a chapter on "The Pulse" in his *Recent Advances in Physiology*.

This assignment brought Lewis and Sir James Mackenzie together, over the latter's "polygraph," and thus began a most useful collaboration; Lewis was twenty-six years of age when he fell under the spell of Mackenzie. Recognizing the need for more exact techniques for recording the electrical phenomena occurring in the heart, Lewis personally acquired an Einthoven string galvanometer and set it up in the basement of University College Hospital. He began with an analysis of auricular fibrillation—a state already produced experimentally by his friend Cushny.

At the age of twenty-nine Lewis wrote his now famous book *The Mechanism of the Heart Beat*. By age thirty-three he was giving the Harvey Lecture in New York. In the field of medical journalism Lewis had launched *Heart* in 1909. He edited it until 1933, at which time it evolved into *Clinical Science*. He edited this, in turn, until 1944—surely a record in bringing up one's brainchild.

With the outbreak of war in 1914 Lewis sought to join a Welsh hospital which was proceeding to Mesopotamia. He was intercepted, however, and finally was convinced by the Medical Research Council that his contribution lay in the field of the "soldier's heart" and the "effort syndrome." His unremitting work at University College Hospital, Hampstead and Colchester was recognized when he was made C.B.E. in 1920 and was knighted in 1921.

Lewis gave up the little practice which he permitted himself and plunged into further work on auricular flutter and fibrillation, with his resultant publications on "circus movement" in the electrical conduction in the heart. Gradually his Harveian outlook brought him into a new field, that of the blood vessels of the human skin, dermatographia and Raynaud-like diseases. From these he shifted to peripheral vascular problems such as ischemia, and thence to pain, and finally to "referred pain." In all, he wrote two hundred and thirty scientific papers and twelve monographs and textbooks. It is little wonder that he had the first of several coronary incidents at age forty-six.

Like Osler, "Tom Lewis," was a shy man, a photographer of birds, a naturalist "strayed into medicine." He was the first Beit Research Fellow, the first full-time professor appointed by the Medical Research Council of Great Britain. He not only trained a generation numbering Parkinson, Paul White and J. C. Meakins, he so built that there will be succeeding generations of research workers produced in the hospitals of the United Kingdom. He believed in young men dedicated to clinical investigation and he laid the groundwork for a brilliant succession of workers in human disease.

Like everyone who pioneers, Lewis had his detractors who felt that he took his self-assigned role of accoucheur to "clinical science" in Britain too seriously. Others poked fun at him by hanging the well-known American picture "The Doctor" in University College Hospital, re-labelled "Clinical Nescience." Some seized upon the endowment of his laboratory and clinical facilities at University College Hospital by the Rockefeller Foundation as further proof that what Lewis advocated was, in fact, some exotic import called "research."

Of course these dying gasps by "the frog men" among physiologists and the high-hatted among clinicians betrayed an inability to comprehend the fact that scientific measurements could be made on human beings who were ill. As Paul White says, Lewis will be remembered for "the links he created between physiological knowledge and technique, and the medical clinic." Just as Richard Bright, through the exclusive use of two wards for one summer at Guy's Hospital had produced his classical work on nephritis, so Lewis, by concentrating heart cases and a suitable recording armamentarium in his ward-laboratory was able to run to earth some of the most important afflictions of the cardiovascular system.

Once he established to his own satisfaction the fact that patients could be studied, not alone for themselves, but as physiological subjects, he embarked upon the equally difficult problem of establishing full-time research as a career, not for himself but for others who would follow. Sir Henry Dale has discussed this aspect of Lewis' life with such completeness that nothing need be added here, save to say that history has proven Lewis right a hundred times over. Today, not only in Britain, but in many parts of the world, the clinical research worker can look forward to a career which is respected, though not often adequately financed.

Lewis would seem, therefore, in retrospect to represent the feeling which came out of the First World War—that clinical science, broadly interpreted, had a contribution to make. Banting and Best in Canada, and Minot and his group in the United States may be mentioned as proof of this thesis, long propounded by Osler. The Second World War proved the sanity and urgency of Lewis' other belief—that clinical science *must* be given the means with which to make its contribution if we are to free ourselves of the sheer waste which disease represents. To select but one example, one might mention the work of Fleming and Florey on penicillin.

The great factor still missing, however, in a world embarrassed by research funds on a temporary or annual basis, is a supply of "home bases," properly financed as permanent research enterprises. The easy problems are gone. Researchers cannot produce a "cure" in one season, let alone a "clue" therein. Any serious clinical research problem is likely to require at least a five-year run, the reason being that the ready applications of basic knowledge have largely been made. Because the recent war's demands were for "applied physiology," the siphoning off of the reservoir of basic physiology has proceeded to a critical level. The call now is to replenish and expand those basic disciplines which have yielded so much of value to clinical investigators. The problem of providing financially for "Tom Lewis' men," wherever they are to be found, is being approached in a number of ways, and nowhere better than in his own country. The lack of these permanent "home bases" still remains, however, the nub of the recruitment problem in medical research.

Tom Lewis, as his students affectionately and universally called him, held advanced ideas on medical education and was sympathetic to students' problems. He was one of the most respected Fellows of the Royal Society. Meakins has given us the following human portrait of him:

> His smile of approbation made the sun shine even through a London fog made worse by working in a photographic dark room in a cellar. . . . Pain to Lewis was not just a symptom of common design. To him it told a story which could only be understood by knowing its language. This could only be written in the last analysis by man—the sufferer. Its many features were as an alphabet—the periodicity, the intensity, the radiation, the quality, the presence of tenderness, and many other features had to be understood and estimated. To him it was not only the commonest of all symptoms but the most informative and elusive.

PLATE 3

(a) Raynaud's illustration of gangrenous toes, in his graduation thesis of 1862. From: Major, Ralph: *Classic Descriptions of Disease*. Courtesy of Charles C Thomas, Publisher.

(b) Christopher Wren's drawing of the arterial Circle of Willis at the base of the human brain. From: Sinclair, H. M. and Robb-Smith, A. H. T.: *A Short History of Anatomical Teaching in Oxford.* Courtesy of The Keeper of Printed Books, Bodleian Library, Oxford.

(c) Jan Swammerdam's composite drawing in his inaugural dissertation *De Respiratione*, 1667. From: Stirling, W.: *Some Apostles of Physiology*, London, 1902.

(d) A. V. Waller's undergraduate illustration of the capillaries in the tongue of the frog. From: Stirling, W.: *Some Apostles of Physiology*, London, 1902.

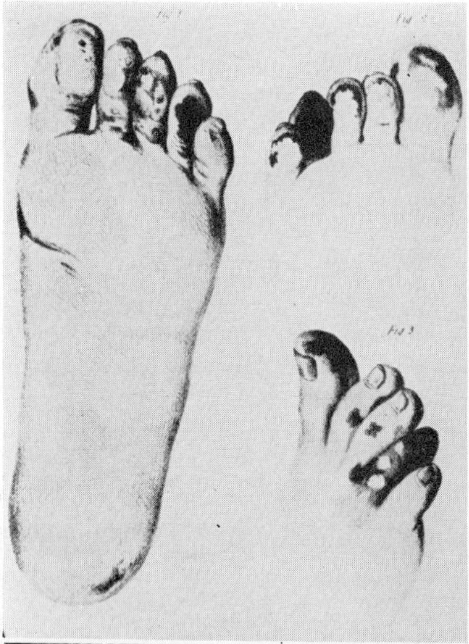

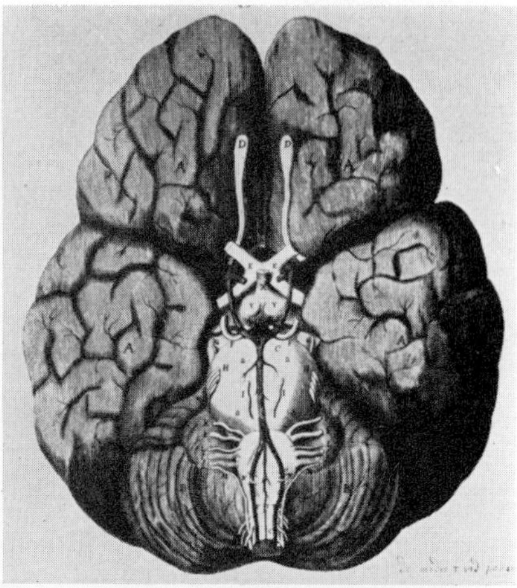

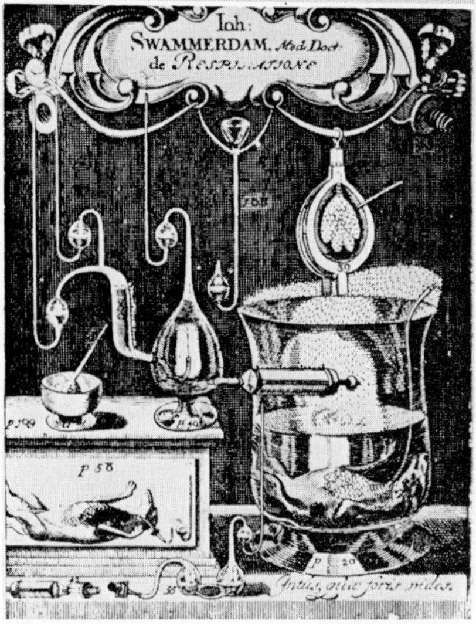

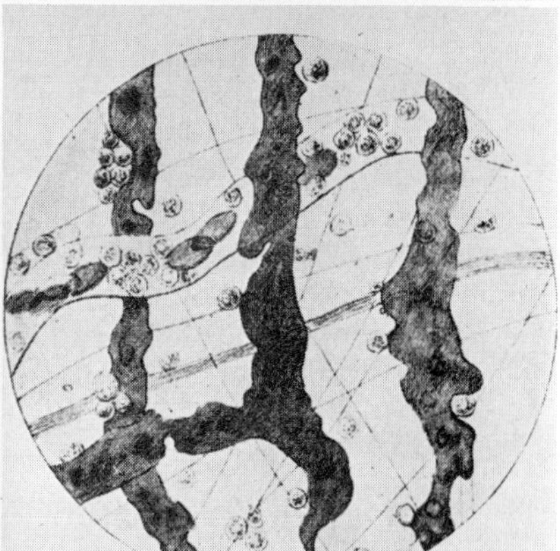

COPY OF A. WALLER'S ORIGINAL FIGURE ON DIAPEDESIS.

←

Chapter V

Chemistry

Joseph Black (1728-1799)

"There is perhaps no other instance of a graduation thesis so weighted with significant novelty as Black's."

—Osler

JOSEPH BLACK was the son of an Irish wine merchant who lived in Bordeaux—the home of the great physiologist, François Magendie. At the age of twelve Joseph was sent home to grammar school in Belfast, and at the age of eighteen he entered the University of Glasgow. Upon the completion of his premedical studies he enrolled in the medical faculty of the University of Edinburgh in 1751.

The rival views of two of his professors, Alston and Whytt, on the treatment of kidney stones, intrigued Black, and in the second year of his course he approached his teacher William Cullen with a plan of investigation. In simplest terms, Black was seeking a treatment for kidney stones which would be superior to the then used lime water. Cullen welcomed him. As Professor Robinson has stated it: "No professor took a more lively interest in the progress of an emulous student than Doctor Cullen. It was his delight to encourage and assist their efforts, and therefore he was not long in attaching Mr. Black to himself, in his most intimate cooperation."

Black commenced work on magnesia alba and it was in heating this substance that he discovered that it lost "a remarkable proportion of its weight in the fire." This fact was more important to him than any cure for kidney stones and thereafter his "attempts were directed to the investigation of this volatile part."

At this distance in time it is hard for us to appreciate the significance of Black's work on carbon dioxide. The gas had been named "gas sylvestre" by van Helmont a century earlier, because it could be produced by burning wood. But now Black appeared with something more than a name for the substance—he called it "fixed air"—he derived it in such a manner that he sounded the death knell of the traditional "phlogiston theory." That theory held that when a substance was heated something was added to it. Black, by using a fine balance—and thus starting quantitative chemical analysis—proved that substances when heated lost weight! Taking lime as an example, he heated it, driving off carbon dioxide or "fixed air."

Black showed this gas to be incapable of supporting life. He knew also that the expired air from animals contained his "fixed air." He wrote:

> Quicklime therefore does not attract air when in its most ordinary form, but is capable of being joined to one particular species only which is dispersed through the atmosphere either in the shape of an exceedingly subtle powder, or more probably in that of an elastic fluid. To this I have given the name of "fixed air."

Black's undergraduate work dating from 1752 was embodied in his graduation thesis *De humore acido a cibis orto, et magnesia alba* which was presented to the Medical Faculty in Edinburgh on June 11, 1754. It was read in amplified form before the Medical Society of Edinburgh on June 5, 1755, and published in 1756 under the title *Experiments upon Magnesia Alba, Quicklime, and some other alkaline substances.* It was twice reprinted, in 1777 and 1782.

Black's later description of these years full of discoveries is interesting. He wrote:

> Here a new and boundless field seemed to open before one. We know not how many different airs may be thus contained in our atmosphere, nor what may be their separate properties. This particular one has evidently very curious and important ones. . . . I fully intended to make this air and some other elastic fluid the subject of serious study. A load of new official duties was laid upon me (i.e. he was elected Professor of Medicine and Chemistry of the University of Glasgow in 1756.) In the same year, however, in which my first account of these experiments was published . . . I had discovered that this particular kind of air, attracted by alkaline substances, is deadly to all animals. . . . And I convinced myself that the change produced on wholesome air by breathing it consisted chiefly, if not solely, in the conversion of part of it into fixed air. For I found, that by blowing through a pipe into lime water, or a solution of caustic alkali, the lime was precipitated and the alkali was rendered mild. . . . In the same year I found that fixed air is the chief part of the elastic matter which is formed in liquids in vinous fermentation. Van Helmont had indeed said this, and it was to this that he first gave the name *gas sylvestre*.

Black's essay on "fixed air" has been classed by some as approaching Newton's *Optics* as a model for investigators. He is still a model for investigators. He is also known for his discovery of "latent heat" and his theory of "specific heat" which provided the basis for the later discoveries and generalizations of Mayer, Joule and Helmholtz in thermodynamics.

As a great and sympathetic teacher Black was widely known. Among his pupils he numbered James Watt of the steam engine, who never failed to acknowledge the training he had received from Black. The medical student-poet, Oliver Goldsmith, also studied with Black. As we shall see presently, Daniel Rutherford, another pupil, was to discover nitrogen while still an undergraduate.

In 1766 Black succeeded to the Chair of Chemistry at Edinburgh, and retired in 1797, a beloved and revered teacher. He died in 1799, as Stirling relates, while eating his frugal meal at the table. He was found by his servant "with his cup—which contained milk diluted with water—on his knees which were joined together, and kept it steady with his hand in the manner of a person perfectly at ease."

Daniel Rutherford (1749-1819)

Daniel Rutherford was born in Edinburgh, November 3, 1749, the son of Dr. John Rutherford, one of the founders of the Edinburgh Medical School. Daniel graduated in Arts at Edinburgh and then embarked on a medical course there, graduating in 1772. After extensive study and travel on the Continent he took up practice in Edinburgh, where he became President of the Royal College of Physicians. In 1786 he succeeded Dr. John Hope in the Chair of Botany. He died at the age of seventy, having long suffered from gout.

As a medical undergraduate Rutherford was attracted to Joseph Black's laboratory where he was given the problem of finding what remained of the atmosphere after combustion, followed by absorption of the "fixed air" thus produced. Seventeen years after Black had presented his graduation thesis on "fixed air," Rutherford published his graduation essay, "Dissertatio Inauguralis de aëre fixo dicto, aut mephitico," thus anticipating Priestley's work.

Rutherford's method, basically, was to remove the oxygen from a sample of air by the burning of charcoal, phosphorus or a candle. He then removed the carbon dioxide with lime or alkali, leaving a residue of what is today known as "nitrogen." The name "nitrogen" was used by the French chemist Chaptal to signify the capacity of this gas to produce nitric acid when electric sparks were passed through it.

Rutherford established the fact also that nitrogen would not support life. He established its exact proportion in air. It is interesting that Lavoisier called this gas "azotic gas" because it would not sustain life.

James Blake (1815-1893)

The discovery of gold in California brought together restless and colourful figures from all parts of the world, none more so than Dr. James Blake. Born in Gosport, England, on July 14, 1815, his education in the medical field was pursued at University

College, London, and probably in France also, for his early publications mention the use of instruments obtained in Paris. Throughout his life he was an admirer of Claude Bernard.

At University College he studied under Thomas Graham and the great physiologist William Sharpey who was to inspire other undergraduate contributors such as Joseph Lister. In 1838, at the age of twenty-three, Blake, the medical student, read a paper before the British Association on the effects of certain salts on the body's metabolism. It was published a year later in the *Edinburgh Medical and Surgical Journal.* This student paper is indeed a milestone. In it Blake recounts what must have been the first determinations on the circulation time of the blood. The burden of his communication was the physiological effect of intra-arterial and intravenous injection into animals, of various chemicals, including strychnine and the recently isolated alkaloids, morphine and nicotine. He published this work in French after communicating it to the Academy of Sciences in Paris. In addition to his theory that the effect produced by drugs was determined by their chemical structure, he proved that drugs act on tissues after reaching them.

He saw his experiments as shedding light in two directions by showing (a) what physiological reactions followed certain chemical injections, and (b) what physico-chemical properties of the reacting tissues might be deduced from the results.

Also, while a senior medical student in 1839 Blake experimented with the obliteration of veins in animals, and communicated his results to the Editor of the Lancet in a discussion of the treatment of varicose veins. He wrote:

> By arresting the circulation in the vessel for a few hours (twelve to sixteen); by passing a couple of needles under it and using the twisted suture; and by the application of gentle external pressure, the slight degree of irritation thus produced will be sufficient to cause such an effusion of lymph and serum in the sheath of the vessel as to lead to its permanent obliteration.

While Blake practised medicine in Conduit Street and Pall Mall in London and qualified as a Fellow of the Royal College of Surgeons, his interests were largely centred on the line of thought of his undergraduate researches. By 1846 he had come to three important conclusions: (a) that the electro-positive element of an injected salt was the determining factor in the resultant physiological reactions; (b) that an increase in toxicity paralleled an increase in the atomic weight of the electro-positive element in inorganic compounds; and (c) that the effects attributable to the electro-positive elements reappear as one ascends the scale of atomic weights. He thought, too, that crystal structure was concerned in these physiological effects. Valence was thought to determine the direction and range of action, with monovalent elements acting specifically on the pulmonary circulation, divalent on the heart, and the higher valences on the central nervous system.

Blake showed that the electro-negative elements, also, could be arranged in order of their physiological reactions. His grouping of all the elements tested is remarkably similar to that developed twenty years later by Mendeljeff in his "Periodic Table."

The restless and skeptical mind of Blake drove him to seek the Western plains of the United States and we find him in 1847 as Professor of Anatomy and Surgery at the St. Louis University Medical College. He wrote on abnormal distribution of the thyroid arteries and on filaria in dogs' hearts. By 1850 he had reached Sacramento, California, where he set up in practice near the busy wharves and undoubtedly treated the miners as they passed into the gold country. By 1856 he was contributing articles on diphtheria and on gun-shot wounds to California's first medical journal. In 1860 he wrote on the ineffectual drug therapy of pulmonary tuberculosis, and quoted his own cases who had gained more from his prescription of rest, sunshine and fresh air. This was twenty years before recognized authorities in the field proposed just such a method!

In 1861 Blake moved to San Francisco, becoming editor of the *Pacific Medical and Surgical Journal* and Professor of Midwifery and Diseases of Women and Children in the Toland Medical College, later the Medical School of the University of California. He served as President of the California Academy of Science for four years and delved into all manner of analyses on drinking waters, ores, fishes and grapes. He believed that grapes which had the highest organic acid and aldehyde content would make the best wine. He also interested himself in the geology of California and Nevada, in local anthropology and in earthquakes. He set up a meteorological station in the Sierra Mountains and one in Southern California and put forward some very original hypotheses based on his recordings. He eventually returned to his researches on chemical composition as related to physiological effects, but in 1876 threw it all up to open a tuberculosis sanitarium in the Mount Saint Helena area of California, not far from the Toll House in which Robert Louis Stevenson and his bride lived after their marriage in San Francisco.

Four years later he gave up his hospital and moved to Middletown, California, where he began spectroscopic studies to further extend his chemico-physiological thesis. He travelled to Europe to present his work in England, France and Germany. One of his communications concerned the toxicity of thallium compounds.

The versatility of this physician may have proved his undoing, but he has most surely been overlooked by medical historians when they have been apportioning credit for the discovery of systems like the "Periodic Table," and for the supposedly modern rest and fresh air treatment of tuberculosis. His medical student interest in "biochemorphology," to use Leake's term, remained with him until the time of his death, in 1893.

Alfred Smee (1818-1877)

Plaster of Paris bandages for splinting injured limbs have been known to medical students for just over a century. The forerunners of these surgical aids were splints composed of chalk and gum devised by a London medical student Alfred Smee. He was a very gifted undergraduate and in 1840, the year in which he qualified to practise medicine, he also published a very fundamental book, *The Elements of Electro-Metallurgy*. For his work in this field he was made a Fellow of the Royal Society in the following year, at the age of twenty-three.

One wonders how this medical student found the time, and especially the space, in which to carry on such large-scale experiments as he did. The fact is that he did this work not in any university setting, but within the walls of the Bank of Engand! How "The Old Lady of Threadneedle Street" came to house such bizarre affairs has been told by J. A. Giuseppi, the archivist of the Bank of England, in his account of "Families of Long Service at the Bank of England." *

Alfred Smee was the son of the distinguished Chief Accountant, William Smee, who resided in the vast premises of the Bank. On the recommendation of the surgeon, Sir Astley Cooper, the recently graduated Alfred Smee was made the first surgeon to the Bank, and spent some of his time in attending porters and clerks of the staff. In 1842 he developed the famous ink known as "Bank Black" which is still used for the writing of the Court Minute Books in England. Twelve years later he joined with others of the Bank staff in introducing a new system of printing bank notes and cheques. He was all his life an innovator and even in his retirement in Surrey carried on an experimental garden.

Paul Ehrlich (1854-1915)

Paul Ehrlich's name is known alike to chemists, bacteriologists and clinicians as a great contributor in these fields of science. Rarely is it appreciated, however, that his prophetic discoveries in the chemistry of tissues and their staining reaction and the associated fields of blood diseases, immunity and bacteriology, actually began during his undergraduate period in medicine.

Ehrlich was born on March 14, 1854 in Upper Silesia, into a prosperous Jewish family. His father was an innkeeper who loved cigars. His mother was a woman with great organizing ability. Any scientific interest in his family setting might be said to stem from his grandfather, who, in the fashion of those times, cultivated an interest in popular science.

In one field at least, Paul Ehrlich might be said to be precocious. At the age of eight he set the town chemist to compound cough-drops to his own boyish prescription. Paul was sent to school in Breslau, where his interest in chemistry was so stimulated that he brought home many ideas and problems to be worked out in the vacations, in the laundry of his home. He had also in school a very good record in Latin. One of the early scientific influences was undoubtedly that of his cousin, Karl Weigert, who was nine years his senior.

* *Genealogists' Magazine, 10:*12, 1949.

After one term at the University of Breslau, Ehrlich moved to the University of Strasbourg, where the famous Professor Waldeyer was just beginning to introduce chemistry into medical studies as a special discipline. With the early development of the German aniline dye industry, Ehrlich had a ready supply of staining agents to apply to tissues. Waldeyer encouraged this early interest of Ehrlich and permitted him to work in his laboratory after the classes were over for the day. It was here that Ehrlich discovered the new type of cell which he called a "mast cell." Having completed his basic sciences, Ehrlich returned to Breslau on Karl Weigert's advice and was there given space to work in the laboratories of the famous Cohnheim and Heidenhain. It is interesting that one of the visitors to the laboratory was Robert Koch, who was in Breslau lecturing on the anthrax bacillus.

At the age of twenty-three and while still an undergraduate, Ehrlich published in the *Archives of Microscopic Anatomy* an outline of his theory of histological staining. He was preoccupied throughout with the "idea of a chemical binding of heterogeneous substances to the protoplasm." This concept he developed into his famous side-chain theory which he exploited during the rest of his life. The facility with which Ehrlich was able to conjure up a three-dimensional picture of the arrangement of the atoms in a particular molecule was undoubtedly one of his greatest assets. As he said, "I can picture the chemical formulae in my mental vision and I believe that this fact has been of the greatest value to me in my studies." Of his earliest childhood, this vivid visual imagery had been a noticeable characteristic.

When Ehrlich graduated at Leipzig with his M.D. degree in 1878 at the age of twenty-four, his thesis was an amplification of his undergraduate work. It was entitled: "Contributions to the Theory and Practice of Histological Staining. Part 1, the Chemical Conception of Staining. Part 2, the Aniline Dyes from Chemical, Technological and Histological Aspects."

Having passed his State Examination as a physician soon afterwards, Ehrlich began as an assistant and later as a senior house physician at the Charité Hospital, Berlin, in the service of Professor von Frerichs. This most sympathetic Chief encouraged Ehrlich in his staining of blood films and his daily use of the diazo-reaction on the urines to be examined in the clinic. The crudeness of the surroundings which von Frerichs was able to offer for this clinical laboratory work in no way discouraged Ehrlich.

In 1882 Ehrlich heard the distinguished country doctor, Robert Koch, lecture before the Berlin Physiological Society on tuberculosis. After the lecture Ehrlich rushed to his laboratory and set up slides covered with tuberculous sputum. These he stained and left overnight on the laboratory stove, long-since cold. In the morning the charwoman in the laboratory started the fire, which so promoted the staining that, when Ehrlich arrived, the tubercle bacilli were everywhere to be seen. On communicating this information and on showing the slides to Robert Koch, the latter became so impressed that he turned his investigations towards the causes underlying the disease rather than to mere descriptions of the effects of tuberculosis.

With von Frerichs' death in 1887, years of hardship and disillusionment began for Ehrlich. The new Chief of the Service, Professor Gerhardt, sought to force Ehrlich into the rigid routine of clinical medicine devoid of any laboratory interest. Ehrlich became depressed and ill and developed tuberculosis. He wisely left Berlin and went to Egypt, where he stayed for two years. There he wrote "When I felt so miserable during the time with Gerhardt, I often stood before the cupboard in which my collection of dyes was stored and said to myself 'These are my friends which will not desert me.'" On returning to Berlin in 1889, Ehrlich was invited by Robert Koch to join him in the new Robert Koch Institute for Infectious Diseases. Here again, Ehrlich's great ability to analyze tissue constituents or foreign substances in tissues, through the use of dyes, brought great reward. He sought to develop chemicals which would attach themselves to bacteria in such a way that the bacteria would be immobilized or killed, and thus laid the groundwork for chemotherapy. He developed the standards which we still use for measuring diphtheria antitoxin in units.

His later discoveries in the field of chemotherapy against syphilis are too well-known to require repetition here. It is remarkable how consistently the threads of Ehrlich's undergraduate studies on blood, lead poisoning, and histological staining with aniline dyes run through all his life's work. The therapeutic vistas opened by this kindly, unworldly and absent-minded professor know no parallel in recent times.

On his death, *The Times* of London carried the following obituary notice: "The vast number of problems he set himself bears witness to the strength of his imagination. He opened 'new doors to the unknown' and the whole world at this hour is his debtor."

Sir Frederick Gowland Hopkins (1861-1947)

Frederick Gowland Hopkins was born at Eastbourne, June 20, 1861. His father died when Frederick was a small child. He was privately educated up to the age of seventeen, when he took his first paid job as a clerk in an insurance office. He did not particularly like the work and stayed for only six months. He then served as an assistant in a commercial analytical laboratory. He has written of this time: "These years taught me something perhaps which might not have been learned elsewhere, for instance, how to obtain results in the shortest possible time; intellectually, they were nearly sterile years."

Hopkins became restless in this atmosphere and as a result undertook to attend a course of lectures at the Royal School of Mines. He was fortunate enough to hear two or three lectures on chemistry from the elder Frankland, which, as Hopkins says, were "the only lectures on chemistry to which I have ever listened." After completing this course, Hopkins joined Dr. P. F. Frankland in a new private laboratory, remaining there only six months, again because of the routine nature of things. Through attendance at the University College, London he prepared himself to pass the examinations required for candidates for the Institute of Chemistry. Having thus come to the notice of Sir Thomas Stevenson, who was a medical expert to the Home Office, Hopkins was invited to become his assistant in a laboratory devoted to medical jurisprudence at Guy's Hospital. In this laboratory Hopkins was able to earn his living while at the same time studying for the medical qualification of the University of London. Once started in medicine he never turned back and his intellectual curiosity was greatly stimulated by each successive phase of the medical course. Though his undergraduate studies kept him hard-pressed for time, he nevertheless did his best to "keep some sort of research going."

Hopkins had already become a contributor to scientific journals and at the age of seventeen published an article in *The Entomologist* dealing with the bombardier beetle. In 1889 while working in the analyst's laboratory he published a report on the chemistry of the pigments in the English brimstone butterfly. This communication was later amplified and the pigments discussed in detail in the Philosophical Transactions of the Royal Society. In a way, this work was the starting point for much of Hopkins' future research on nitrogenous compounds. He showed that the pigment isolated from the butterfly's wing was a uric acid derivative. Typically, Hopkins came up with an improved method for estimating uric acid, which was later to be the key with which he opened several doors in medical research.

In 1894 he qualified under the Conjoint Board and received his London M.B. degree. In 1898 he was invited to join Sir Michael Foster at Cambridge in the teaching of "chemical physiology," and to assist in research being undertaken in Foster's laboratory. Though he went in fear and trepidation, he remained and spent his very productive life there.

To revert to his work on uric acid estimation, Hopkins became interested in studies of dietary protein and its supposed influence on the amount of uric acid excreted by the body. This led him to experiments on purified proteins to be included in artificial diets. By 1901 he had isolated and identified, with the help of S. W. Cole, the key substance tryptophane. Progressing in the same logical sequence, he, along with Edith G. Willcock, started to work out the nutritionally essential amino acids, showing among other things that zein could be improved upon by the addition of tryptophane. In turn this led to his theory of "unidentified accessory food factors," which were highly essential in any diet, no matter how rich it might be in proteins, carbohydrates, fats and minerals. His interest in pathological physiology then led him to a survey of deficiency diseases arising from a protracted

"I have memory of an address given by him [Sir Frederick Gowland Hopkins] at a British Association meeting. In an uninviting, gaunt lecture-room he decanted for nearly an hour on the cell as the theatre of chemical processes. Without any deliberate attempt at eloquence . . . he conjured up for his audience . . . a picture of the cell as a tiny sponge containing perhaps a thousand foci of different actions cooperatively confined within a unitary whole. An organized factory manifoldly hydrolysing, pulling to pieces, and contemporaneously constructing and reconstructing. And this unity bounded outwardly by a mosaic of countless chemical pores and leaking like a sieve. As I listened I felt I was being privileged for the time to see something of the microcosmic world in which my friend's scientific thoughts took shape and did his bidding. One mental factor which, it seemed to me, such thinking must demand, was a peculiar intensity of visual 'imagination, continuously checked in factual knowledge.' "

—Sir Charles Sherrington in an Obituary Note on F. G. Hopkins.

lack of his "accessory food factors," which we now call vitamins.

In 1929 Hopkins shared the Nobel Prize with Eijkman, well-known for his work on the deficiency disease, beri-beri.

It would be wrong to imply that Hopkins' entire life centred about the discovery of accessory food factors for, in fact, he did pioneer work in many unrelated fields. For instance, he, along with Walter Fletcher, was the first to accurately determine the lactic acid production arising from muscular work. Hopkins was greatly interested in the cell catalyst glutathione, which he believed to be a dipeptide. When Blythe Eagles and Hunter, much younger workers in the field, showed that glutathione was actually a tripeptide, Hopkins set out to improve his method of isolation of the compound and hastened to confirm their results.

Hopkins' work came at an opportune time in the history of cell chemistry, especially in tissue oxidations and in reductive processes. He produced 132 papers in his lifetime, many of them landmarks in biochemistry. He was made a Fellow of the Royal Society in 1905 and became its President in 1931.

This much-beloved teacher became Professor of Biochemistry at Cambridge and Head of the Sir William Dunn Institute of Biochemistry. He was knighted in 1925 and the Order of Merit was conferred upon him in 1935.

With his distinguished white head and his flowing mustache, this slight figure was the most magnetic of men. He did not live isolated from the world, but like Rudolf Virchow, he was part of the world and knew a great deal about it. As early as 1896 he helped to establish in London the Clinical Research Association which offered a pathological service to practitioners and involved a great deal of night work for Hopkins. In his later years and despite his blindness, which was gradually handicapping him, he remained the patron saint of modern biochemistry, ever kind, ever tolerant of youth and ever humble.

No account of Sir Frederick Gowland Hopkins would be complete without a reference to the spirit of the laboratory around him at Cambridge. From 1923-1931 a group of brilliant editors, associated with Hopkins in his biochemical work, produced an amazing annual called *Brighter Biochemistry*. Thus for the year 1924-25 J. B. S. Haldane contributed to this annual a report which commenced:

Sir, on the upper floor the classes
Included genii and asses,
The former got out tryptophane,
The latter poured it down the drain etc.

On the occasion of Hopkins' knighthood, Barnet Woolf produced the accompanying cartoon (Fig. 93).

Hopkins always gave a hand with the comic annual and produced the following masterpiece on "Biochemical Equipment—A Glance into the Future," in which he contrasts the rude equipment of 1898 with that of the present and of the supposed A.D. 2000 version. The 1898 portion of the dialogue between himself, as "Aminophilus," and Sir W. B. Hardy, the colloid expert, as "Collophilus," is reproduced below:

Biochemical Equipment—A Glance into the Future

A.D. 1898.

(A small room in the building which still adorns Corn Exchange Street)

Collophilus: Pray lend me your test tube, Aminophilus; my own is under repair.

Aminophilus: Most certainly, Collophilus; I know that it will receive your customary care in the handling of apparatus. You find me, as it happens, in a philanthropic mood; Charles has just captured a mouse in the cellar.

C: Felicitations. You will at last be able to proceed with your Nutritional Investigations. Let me confess that I, too, am in expansive mood. Before leaving my house this morning, I was able to purloin an egg (I think a fresh one) from the domestic store. I may say that the yolk, and part of the white, are very heartily at your service.

A: Too generous. I am, it is true, in need of a source of amino acids; but nothing must interfere with your important Colloidal Studies.

C: Believe me, it is impossible for me to employ, at the moment, all the material represented by a whole egg. The Laboratory, I find, lacks any source of polyvalent ions. I possess sodium chloride, which, like the egg, is of domestic extraction; but can you, I wonder, provide me with a minimal quantity of, say, ammonium sulphate?

A: Fortunately, owing to the generosity of the Professor of Agriculture, I possess a specimen of that useful salt. A portion is at your command.

C: Encouraging in the very highest degree. You embolden me to mention, though with much hesitation, my need for metallic ions of high valency. I possess a solution of pen-nibs in hydrochloric acid, but—

A: If, my dear Collophilus, you are venturing to think of salts, of, let us say, Cerium or Thallium (I mention them with awe), then indeed you are, as you claim, in expansive mood. We must, you know, be reasonable. May I suggest a possibility? I am thinking of the domestic store. Could you not try alum?

C: An inspiration. Tomorrow the coagulation potency of a trivalent ion shall be explored.

(On the morrow Collophilus opens a new Chapter of Science.)

PLATE 4

(a) Sir Frederick Gowland Hopkins carrying his banner "Gluta thy Owne" as depicted by B. Woolf in, *Hopkins and Biochemistry*. Courtesy of W. Heffer and Sons, Cambridge.

(b) Paul Ehrlich at the age of twenty-four. From: *Paul Ehrlich* by Martha Marquardt, London, William Heinemann Medical Books, Ltd., 1949.

(c) Paul Langerhans at age twenty-six. Courtesy of Dr. Hyman Morrison.

(d) Humphry Davy at the age of twenty-three. Courtesy of the Royal Institution, London.

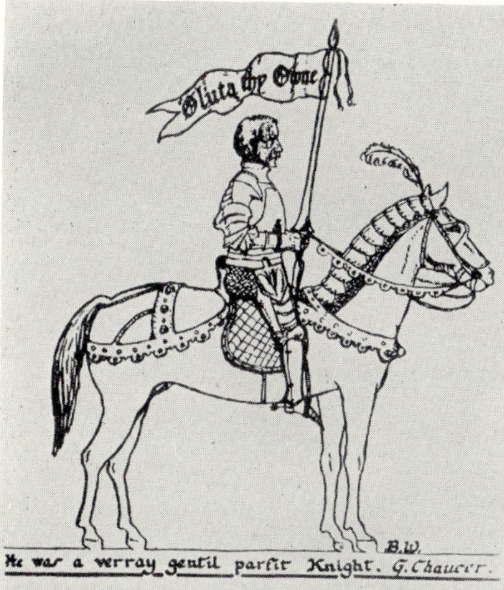

Cartoon on the occasion of Sir F. G. Hopkins' Knighthood, by B. Woolf.

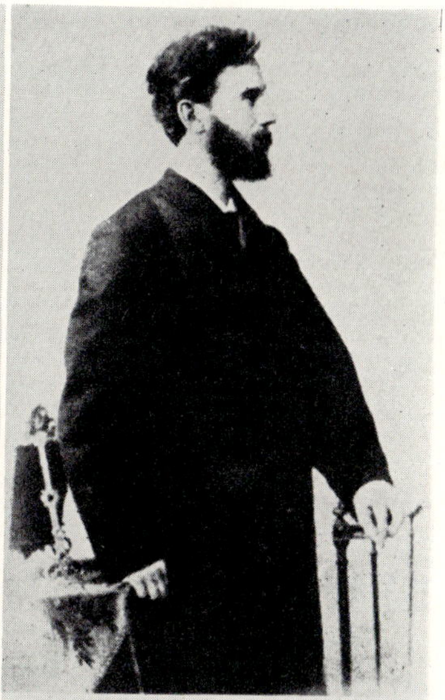

Paul Ehrlich aged twenty-four

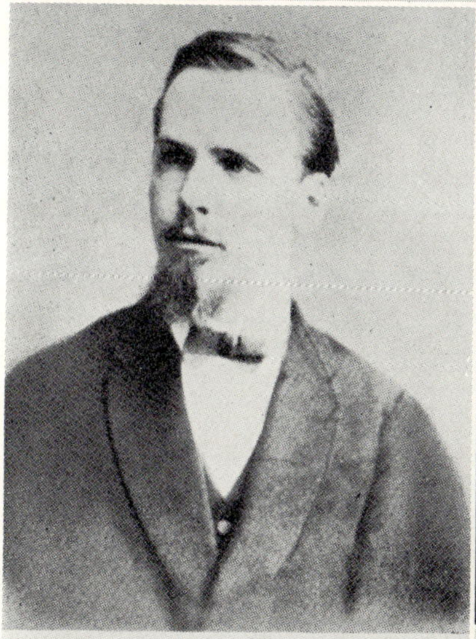

PAUL LANGERHANS 1873

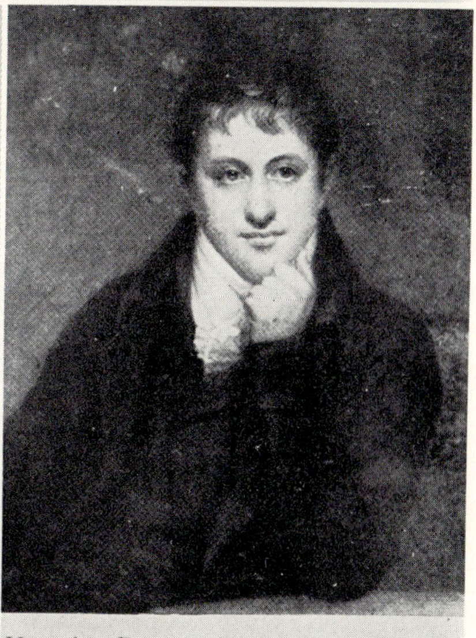

Humphry Davy at the age of twenty-three
From the painting by H. Howard

Chapter VI

Digestion

THE STORY of the study of man's digestive processes is replete with the names of student contributors. In this chapter we shall consider Stensen, de Graaf, J. R. Young, Claude Bernard, Pavlov and W. B. Cannon.

Niels Stensen (Steno) (1638-1686)

Niels Stensen was the son of the Court Jeweller in Copenhagen, who died unfortunately when his son was six years of age. Raised by his grandparents Stensen had a private tutor who taught him Latin, German, Dutch, French, Italian, English, Hebrew and Greek. At Grammar School he came under the benevolent influence of Ole Borch whose interests ranged from medicine and natural science to chemistry and philology, and whose proficiency was to lead him to a Chair in the University.

At the age of eighteen Stensen entered the University after a boisterous initiation ceremony. He chose as his preceptor Thomas Bartholin, the famed anatomist. Stensen had been at University two years when the armies of Sweden overran Denmark and laid siege to Copenhagen. The student regiment, 266 strong, took its place on the barricades, with Stensen as a corporal in charge of 86 of them. Twice in the eighteenth and twice in the nineteenth century students were called to defend their beautiful and cultured city. In Stensen's day it was the Dutch fleet which broke the siege and ended the famine.

It is not surprising therefore that Bartholin should send his pupil to Amsterdam to continue his undergraduate medical studies under his friend Blasius. It was in his laboratory on April 7, 1661, that Stensen made his first great discovery. He had purchased a sheep's head for dissection and was working on the veins of the face when, to his surprise, his scalpel slipped through a "cavity" and struck the teeth with a metallic sound. Stensen had really been working inside the duct which leads the saliva of the parotid gland into the mouth. This we still call Stensen's duct.

Blasius dismissed this as a freak of nature, and explained patiently to Stensen that the true function of the parotid gland was to warm the ear! Then he pretended to have known about the parotid duct for years, so that Stensen, having confirmed the existence of the duct in the dog also, moved on, wisely, to Leyden to work with Sylvius and van Horne. There in July, 1661, he gave his famous "Disputation" on his discovery. Within a short time Stensen discovered the duct of the lachrymal gland, the ducts of the sublingual gland and the buccal glands, thus adding to his student reputation.

In 1662 he published his findings in *Observationes Anatomicae.* Two years later, in Copenhagen, he published his "De musculis et glandulis observationum specimen," dedicated to King Friedrich III. He propounded the theory that the glandular secretion was manufactured in the glands themselves and was secreted through the ducts. He discovered the follicles in the ovaries, and "Peyer's" patches of the intestine.

Concerning the muscles Stensen's views created a sensation second only to that which followed Harvey's publication of 1628. He wrote: "The heart has been considered the seat of natural warmth, as the throne of the soul and even as the soul itself. Some have greeted the heart as the sun, others as the King; but if you examine it more closely, one finds it to be nothing more than muscle."

Stensen travelled to Paris where he addressed Thevenot's circle of savants (including Swammerdam) in a most remarkable dis-

"Gentlemen,

Instead of promising that I shall satisfy your curiosity in what relates to the Anatomy of the Brain, I begin by publickly and frankly owning that I know nothing of the matter. I wish I were the only Person under the necessity of talking in this manner, because I might in time become acquainted with what others know; and it would be a great blessing to Mankind if this most delicate Part, and which is liable to so many dangerous Diseases, were as well understood as the generality of Anatomists and Philosophers imagine it to be. In this, few imitate the Sincerity of Sylvius who never talks positively concerning the Brain, though he has been at more pains about it than any man that I know. The number of those who think everything easy is infinitely the greatest; and they give us the History of the Brain and Disposition of its Parts with the same confidence and assurance, as if they had been present at the Formation of this surprising Machine, and had been let into all the Designs of the Great Architect. Though the number of these positive Gentlemen be very great, and though I cannot pretend to answer for the Sentiments of all the rest, I am nevertheless very much convinced that they who search for solid Knowledge will find nothing satisfactory in all that has been written about the Brain. It is very certain that it is the principal Organ of the Soul and the Instrument by which it works very wonderful Effects. The Soul which imagines it can penetrate into everything without it; and that nothing in the World can set bounds to its Knowledge, is nevertheless utterly at a loss to describe its own Habitation, and is nowhere more to seek than at home. We need only view a Dissection of that large Mass, the Brain, to have ground to bewail our Ignorance. On the very Surface you see varieties which deserve your admiration; but when you would look into its inner Substance you are utterly in the dark, being able to say nothing more than that there are two Substances one greyish the other white, which last is continuous with the Nerves distributed all over the body; that the greyish Substance serves in some places for a Cortex to the White, and that in other places it separates the white Filaments from each other.

If we are asked what these Substances are in what manner the Nerves are joined in the white Substance or how far their Extremities penetrate into it; all we can do is to own our ignorance, except we be resolved to increase the number of those who prefer the applause of the publick to sincerity and truth. For, to say that the white Substance is only an uniform Body like Wax without any Art concealed in it, would be to think too meanly of this great Masterpiece of Nature. We are sure that wherever there are Fibres in the Body, they always observe a certain regular order more or less complex in proportion to the Functions for which they are appointed. If this Substance is everywhere Fibrous, as it appears in many places to be, you must own that these Fibres are disposed in the most artful manner; since all the diversity of our Sensations and Motions depends upon them. We admire the contrivance of the Fibres of every Muscle, and ought still more to admire their disposition in the Brain, where an infinite number of them contained in a very small Space, do each execute their particular Offices without confusion or disorder."

(From "Dissertation on the Anatomy of the Brain" by Nicolas Stensen, read in the Assembly held in M. Thevenot's house in the year 1665 in Paris. Translation by Professor E. Busch.)

course on the brain. This was published in the work of his grand-nephew Winslow, "Exposition anatomique de la structure du corps humain." Recently the distinguished Danish neurosurgeon Edward Busch has translated this discourse into English from which the attached extracts are taken.

Doubtless under the patronage of Thevenot, Stensen visited Italy, and in Florence, with the backing of Viviani, Galileo's biographer, was appointed physician to Ferdinand II, Grand Duke of Tuscany, a patron of the sciences. Stensen was given a pension, a residence and a connection with the ancient Hospital of Santa Maria Nuova, founded in 1288. At least in Florence Stensen had more opportunities for work than Vesalius had enjoyed in Madrid!

In Florence Stensen was converted to Catholicism. Five years later, King Christian V of Denmark asked him to return as Professor of Geology, a subject in which he had developed a great interest in Italy. In fact he is regarded as the father of scientific geology. Once home in Denmark, however, he became embroiled in religious differences and after two years left to become a Bishop in Germany. He died in the service of the Church in 1686.

An echo of Stensen's student work comes to us in Albrecht von Haller's graduation thesis in 1728 at Leyden wherein the erroneous view of Coschwitz, the surgeon and professor of anatomy at Halle, that the lingual vein was the true duct of the submaxillary gland, was disproved by this brilliant student.

Regnier de Graaf (1641-1673)

Our next contributor in the study of digestion was Regnier de Graaf. He was born in the town of Schoonhaven, which lies between Rotterdam and Arnheim. His father was a man of keen intellect and was interested in architecture and in the development of hydraulic machines. De Graaf embarked upon the study of medicine at Utrecht under van Diemerbroeck whom he called "An excellent professor to whom I owe the progress I have made in the study of the human body." During the year 1663, de Graaf transferred to the University of Leyden where he studied under such stimulating teachers as John van Horne and François de la

Böe (Sylvius). He was a contemporary of the students Stensen, Frederick Ruysch and Jan Swammerdam.

In 1664, at the age of 23, de Graaf published his first scientific work, the preparation of which had occupied a considerable amount of his time as a medical student. It was entitled "Disputatio medica de natura et usu succi pancreatici." It was ninety pages in length and contained three excellent plates, describing his method of collecting pancreatic juice by a temporary fistula. Two hundred years later another student, Claude Bernard, was to re-discover this long-neglected procedure. The book began with a dedication to his father, to relatives and to the senators and councillors of Schoonhaven. Looking back on his early trials as a student researcher, he later said, "After racking the brain and putting the spirit to all sorts of torture to find a proof that would completely satisfy us, we found a method by the grace of God." The method, which worked so successfully, employed the quill of a wild duck which he states to have been longer and thinner than that of any other bird. He fashioned a small retractable wooden plug on a thread to be passed through the hollow of the quill until it stopped up the narrow distal orifice. Taking a fasting animal, he performed a tracheotomy and opened the abdomen. He tied off the duodenum at the pyloric junction and washed out its contents. He placed the quill in the pancreatic duct and passed the attached thread through a telescoping paper tube which was to conduct the juice to a flask. The flask had an air escape hole in it through which the thread finally passed. When all was in order he pulled the thread and started to collect the precious pancreatic juice. He managed to collect as much as an ounce of the juice in a seven-hour period.

De Graaf canalized the pancreatic duct and the parotid duct simultaneously in one animal in order to show that the two juices were different. He tested the juice by tasting it and noticed periodic variations in its apparent acidity and salinity. Sometimes he classed it as "insipid." At Angers he had an opportunity to dissect out the pancreas of a sailor who had just been killed by a falling mast. He tasted and made other observations on the juice encountered in this case also.

In the fashion of the times, physiological theory far outdistanced observable facts. De Graaf's views on the pancreatic juice largely reflected the teaching of Sylvius who believed that "effervescence" was a main feature of digestion and was parallel in some manner to physiological fermentation.

De Graaf thus listed as the uses of the pancreatic juice (a) the promotion of effervescence with the assistance of the bile, in order to dispose of the mucus inside the intestine. This in turn was to allow the lacteals to absorb the chyle of the digested food; (b) the pancreatic juice had also the important function of separating the usable part of the food from the useless.

A French edition, considerably enlarged, appeared in Paris in 1666, in which de Graaf referred to the works of Stensen, Wirsung, Rudbeck, Bartholin, Wharton, Harvey and others. Bartholin had imagined that the pancreas was the excretory organ of the spleen just as the bile duct was considered the excretory organ of the liver. However, de Graaf disproved this quickly when he splenectomized a dog and later collected pancreatic juice through his temporary fistula.

On July 23, 1665, de Graaf received his Doctor of Medicine degree from the University of Angers. He then travelled in France for a considerable time, never neglecting his anatomical studies. As he says, "In my journeys in France, I put all my energies to the dissection of bodies which I found there in sufficiently great quantities; I preferred most to dissect the pancreas and the genital parts since I found there consistently new things, unremarked by anatomists before me."

For a time in 1666, de Graaf returned to practise in Delft. However, the year 1667 finds him back in Paris as the centre of interest in a coterie collected by Dr. Bourdelot, to whose home, de Graaf records, "the most curious wits of the University do frequently resort." On one occasion de Graaf depancreatized a dog before Dr. Bourdelot's gathering. Though the doctor told his servants to watch the dog carefully, it later succumbed. Two and one half centuries later another young student, Charles Best, working with Frederick Banting, in Toronto, was to learn the reason why.

De Graaf returned to Delft where, in 1668, he published his three remarkable treatises in one volume: "De virorum organis generationi inservientibus"; "De clysteribus"; and "De usu siphonis in anatomia." His hydraulically-minded father had nothing on Regnier de Graaf who used a length of bird's intestine with a quill at either end to permit blood transfusions between animals. The design of syringe developed for anatomical injections, using a silver or copper barrel and a leather plunger, resembles our modern instruments.

In 1672 de Graaf's greatest work was issued. It is that for which he is chiefly famous today. Its title was "De mulierum organis generationi inservientibus." A translation of its sub-title would read, "A new treatise wherein it is demonstrated that man and all those animals that are called vivipara, these no less than the ovipara, derived their origin from the egg."

A year later de Graaf was dead, a victim of the plague, at the age of thirty-two.

His work, "De virorum," established the tubular nature of the testicular tissue. He was at great pains to put down fantastic theories about certain vital elements in the blood being miraculously transferred to these tubules. With his newly invented syringe, he injected the spermatic blood vessels with mercury and showed them to be quite distinct from the semen-bearing tubules. He never discoursed on his anatomical findings without stating the generalization deriving from them. Hence he said, "Man, then, cannot be immortal on this earth, but he has the consolation in dying, of living again in his children, and God has given him the means of generation, not only for a thousand years but even for a species of Eternity—and for this purpose there are certain organs of the human frame fashioned with a structure so delicate that the hand of Providence may therein be witnessed."

The basic and well planned research which preceded his publication of "De Mulierum organis generationi" must excite our admiration today. He has left us excellent drawings of the rapidly developing embryo examined at predetermined times in the best experimental tradition. His supply of experimental animals encompassed one hundred rabbits, forty goats and many other assorted species. In addition to the stages of embryonic development he gave us the first description of the corpus luteum.

De Graaf was ever thorough and called on his former colleagues at Leyden for supplementary proof of his own theories. He wrote: "One can assert that the females of all sorts of animals have eggs, since they are found not only in birds and in oviparus and viviparus fish, but also in quadripeds and in women. We have found eggs in rabbits, hares, pigs, sheep and cows. . . . I begged Stensen to appraise me of his observations in species that I lacked. He did not neglect to reply frankly, saying that he found eggs of different sizes in deer, guinea pigs, badgers, roe deer, wolves and asses; in mules even and in other animals."

In the nine-year period between the publication of his student research on the pancreatic juice and his death in 1673, we find a record of resourceful industry, rarely equalled. The combination of manual dexterity and ability to plan an experiment, of which we saw evidence in his student work, is even better exemplified by his later and greater works on the organs of reproduction and their function.

Two things strike us forcibly from this brief consideration of the works of Regnier de Graaf. First, that it was a time for discovery—with his contemporaries Stensen, Swammerdam and Ruysch all making great names for themselves. Secondly, one sees a common denominator running through the careers of these men—and that is the sagacity and the helpfulness of the great teacher Sylvius. He believed in his students and this belief, as history shows, was fully justified.

Footnote on Digestion

Edward Stevens in 1777 presented a dissertation at Edinburgh for his M.D. degree, "De alimentorum concoctione." Stevens is said to have first isolated the gastric juice and performed digestive experiments outside of the body. Michael Foster in his admirable *History of Physiology* notes that Stevens took advantage "of a man of weak understanding who gained a miserable livelihood by swallowing stones for the amusement of the common people." Stevens was quick to see the investigative possibilities of this man's stomach and had him swallow small perforated spheres made of silver, within which he had wrapped foods both raw and cooked, and even specimens of bone. Forty-eight hours later the spheres were examined after they had been voided, whereupon it was found

→

John Richardson Young (1782-1804)

Our next student pioneer is John Richardson Young from western Maryland, who in 1803 wrote his graduation thesis at the University of Pennsylvania School of Medicine on "An Experimental Inquiry into the Principles of Nutrition and the Digestive Process."

Young opens his essay by rejecting the teachings of William Cullen of Edinburgh which had been that vegetables possessed food value because of their acid content, along with their contained sugar and oil. Young also held that water went into the formation of the body solids. He discussed the association between salivary secretion and gastric juice secretion with great insight.

Young experimented chiefly on animals which swallowed their food without breaking it up by physical means. The large American bullfrog (rana ocellata) was therefore used, and the rates of dissolution of field mice, spring frogs, ground beef and veal, in the frog's capacious and easily-entered stomach, were recorded. Snakes were used also, and into their stomachs a great variety of things was forced, such as lizards and small frogs. Fleshy parts were dissolved and bones and teeth were softened, but only at one half the speed of the process already observed in the bull frog. All food retracted from their stomachs, by threads previously tied to it, showed a red or acidic reaction on litmus paper.

To compare human digestion with that already studied, he swallowed the condyles of the thigh bone of a chicken, and observed their greatly softened state and their weight loss four days later. He also placed in frogs' stomachs little linen bags

←

that whole grains of legumes and wheat were hardly digested at all. Experiments were done on dogs and sheep as well as on oxen, and in the case of the latter animals the vegetable foods were readily digested. Meat of course was not so well digested. From a dog's stomach, however, a fluid was withdrawn which readily digested cooked meat outside of the body without any suggestion of putrefaction. In this, of course, Stevens was answering the long-held theory that digestion was a form of putrefaction. The early American physiologist Young came to the same conclusions. In fact, the views of Stevens and Young were very close to those of the Italian experimenter and philosopher Spallanzani.

Benjamin Rush, while a student at Edinburgh, wrote his thesis on the digestion of food also, and carried out a number of unusual experiments on his own stomach in the process. His degree was granted in June, 1768.

containing bread, peas, beans and wheat. After thirty hours only the bread was gone. The intact peas, beans and wheat had resisted "the gastric menstruum." However, when these were broken up, as they would be by the jaws of animals, Young found them dissolved, after a suitable time in the stomach of the frog. For good measure Young's book even quotes Morgagni's story of a young lady, living on vegetables in Lent, throwing up a fully developed plant "with perfect leaves and roots!"

As further proof that the gastric juice acted with impartiality on animal and vegetable foods, Young cited the relevant literature, mentioning two polar bears who grew fat on a vegetable diet only, and a pigeon which was trained to eat meat, even to the exclusion of grain from its diet.

With ingenious experiments upon himself and upon his bullfrogs he concluded that digestion was not analogous to the fermentation of wine nor the putrefaction of food. His friend Mitchell "avoided his usual breakfast, in the place of which he took, between the hours of eight and ten, twelve ounces of sugar. Nothing more was taken until one o'clock. Having the power to ruminate, it was at this hour thrown up; the mass was sweet . . . no disengagement of air was to be perceived . . . there was not the least eructation of air during the whole period the experiment was going on. If ever a vinous fermentation took place in the stomach, we expected to have found it in this experiment as this viscus was plentifully supplied with saccharine matter, which passes so readily to this state; but as nothing of the kind occurred, we conclude the vinous fermentation has nothing to do with the digestive process."

Against the theory of digestion as putrefaction he wrote: "On an empty stomach I made a light dinner, on chicken pye, and drank simple water; in half an hour, by irritating my fauces, it was thrown up; at this time it was plentifully supplied with gastric fluid, as well as saliva, as the quantity of food was but small. It was then exposed in a tumbler to a heat equal to the human temperature. For the space of nine hours there was not . . . any disengagement of air. As digestion is performed sooner than this period, it was not attended to any longer."

Young was able to place litmus paper in the stomach of a bullfrog which had had no food for two days. On retraction it was coloured red, as by an acid. Young made experiments upon himself, taking meat on an empty stomach. After regurgitating it, he established the fresh and non-putrefied nature of the meat and the acid nature of the juice enveloping it. He concluded: "We have little hesitation, therefore, in saying that the acid so constantly found in the stomach of man, and almost, probably, all animals, is to be referred to their gastric fluid."

The rudimentary chemical methods at hand led Young, incorrectly, to suppose that the acid was phosphoric acid. But the main content of his thesis was first class in every respect. He speculated on the possibility of using gastric juice to dissolve large kidney stones, and even experimented with human kidney stones placed in the stomach of a bullfrog, pulled out and weighed every two days!

Young's attempt to synthesize a theory of digestion to replace that which he had demolished was very thorough. He wrote, in part: "Aliment is dissolved by the gastric menstruum; it then passes into the duodenum and meets with bile and pancreatic liquor; after being united with these, a heterogeneous mass is formed called chyme, and from this the lacteals secrete chyle." He was a good clinical observer too, and mentioned the fact that "nutrition goes on when the biliary ducts are obstructed, and also when the pancreas is scirrhous."

Young was the son of Dr. Samuel Young and Ann Richardson Young of Hagerstown, Maryland. The father, a graduate of Trinity College, Dublin, and an M.D. from Edinburgh, was to live to the age of 108. His wife died, probably of tuberculosis, at 31. Their son died in 1804, one year after graduating in medicine at the University of Pennsylvania. He was not only a good investigator, but a literary man. He had been active in the Cliosophic Literary Society at Princeton University where he graduated in 1799.

Howard Kelly was interested in Young and wrote of his life in the Johns Hopkins Hospital Bulletin: "Young's name will shine with an even brighter luster, as the one who first effectively introduced and patiently followed out in this country the modern laboratory methods. Young was our first real scientist in the field of medicine."

Claude Bernard (1813-1878)

While many of the researches by students already described in this work would seem to concern relatively trivial subjects, such could not be said of the two undergraduate works of Claude Bernard, the father of experimental medicine.

Claude Bernard was born at Saint-Julien (Rhone) near Villefranche, on July 12, 1813, the son of a small estate proprietor and wine grower. The parental farm was so situated that on a clear day one could see the Alps in the distance. Claude Bernard was to use it later as a summer cottage.

The village curé taught the boy music and Latin, until it was time to attend the Jesuit college at Villefranche. After leaving the college Claude Bernard went to Lyons, where he worked for approximately two years as a pharmacist. The quackery and subterfuge which he found in the business there thoroughly sickened him and he gave it up. However, he found time to write a vaudeville comedy, *La Rose du Rhone*, which was performed. In addition, he composed a prose drama, *Arthur de Bretagne*, which was published posthumously in 1886 in Paris.

Armed with these literary works, he set off with two companions for Paris at the age of 21 and sought there the advice of the dramatic critic at the Sorbonne, Saint-Marc Girardin, who advised him to study medicine, despite his talent in the theatre.

The decision made, Claude Bernard threw himself into his studies in anatomy and physiology especially. In order to support himself he opened a course of lectures in a little experimental laboratory, which he set up opposite the Collège de France. Unfortunately it soon closed for lack of students. Bernard was not a distinguished student; in fact he was rather inattentive. This may be accounted for by the numerous serious flaws which he detected in his Professors' lectures. Fortunately, however, in his fifth year he became preparateur to the famous Magendie, Professor of Medicine in the Collège de France, actually occupying Laennec's old chair.

Despite the fact that Bernard had to continue to give private tutoring and lectures in order to cover his student expenses, he pioneered with his little undergraduate researches. By May of

1843 he was ready to publish his first paper describing work which he had done on the distribution of the chorda tympani, his interest having been stimulated by a case of facial hemiplegia which he had seen as a student on the wards. We shall see in his later years an oft-recurring interest in this subject.

In the same year Bernard published his doctoral thesis on his undergraduate researches on gastric juice. His excellent basis in anatomy and great manual dexterity were evident from the thesis. He described his work on the intravenous injection into an animal of cane sugar and of his finding it unchanged in the urine. When, however, it was injected after the contents of a fresh stomach had acted upon it, the sugar recovered in the urine was no longer cane sugar. This was the germ of his later enquiry into the glycogenic function of the liver. The changing of cane sugar into blood sugar by the gastric juice was one of the things which stimulated his life interest in nutrition.

In 1843 also he became interested in the role of the pancreas in digestion, and again his ability as a dissector led him to see that the pancreatic duct entered the gut in almost the same area in which he had noticed the filling of the lacteals in the dog after a meal. To further his studies, he improved upon the pancreatic fistula devised by Regnier de Graaf (1662). He hypothesized a three-fold action of pancreatic juice. This was revolutionary teaching in a world which regarded all digestion as being accomplished by the stomach alone. Bernard set out originally to study carbohydrate metabolism and that of fat and protein as well. His interest in diabetes caused him to begin with the carbohydrates and he never progressed beyond that stage of his plan.

Still turning over in his mind the problem of diabetes, Claude Bernard set himself to find out where the dextrose in the blood was destroyed. His friend, Barreswil the chemist, had just devised the copper sulphate test for dextrose. And with this key Claude Bernard set out on his hunt. He found instead where glucose is produced. He discovered that the hepatic vein carrying blood away from the liver was loaded with glucose, even in a dog fed on meat only and with no sugar in the diet. He then thought of the liver as an organ or gland which "secreted" sugar.

Bernard was faced with the additional theory that the liver

"About 1844 I was studying the digestive powers of gastric juice by the help of the method introduced by Blondlot, namely, that of collecting gastric juice by means of a cannula, or sort of silver tap, fitted into the stomach of a live dog in such a way that the health of the animal does not in the least suffer thereby. Just then the celebrated surgeon of Berlin, Dieffenbach, was on a visit to Paris; and, hearing of my experiments through my friend Pelouze, he was anxious to witness the operation of the introduction of the gastric cannula. Informed of his wish, I hastened to gratify it, and performed the experiment on a dog in the chemical laboratory which Pelouze then had in the Rue Dauphine. After the operation the animal was shut up in the yard of the laboratory in order that we might examine it again later on. But on the morrow it was found that the dog had, in spite of precautions, escaped, carrying still in its belly the accusing cannula of the physiologist. Some days afterwards, quite early in the morning, before I had got up, I was visited by a person who came to tell me that the police commissioner of the quarter of the Ecole-de-Medicine wanted to speak with me, and requested me to call on him. In the course of the day I presented myself at the police office in the Rue du Jardinet. I found there a little old man of a very respectable appearance, who received me coldly, and at first said nothing. Then, taking me into an adjoining room, he showed me, to my great astonishment, the dog on which I had operated in Pelouze's laboratory, and asked me if I admitted having placed in the dog the instrument which he had in his belly. I replied in the affirmative, adding that I was delighted to find my cannula again, for I had given it up as lost. My answer, however, instead of satisfying the commissioner, appeared to anger him, for he addressed to me an admonition couched in the severest terms, accompanied by threats at my audacity in having taken his dog to experiment on. I explained that it was not I who had taken his dog, but that I had bought it off the men who were in the habit of selling dogs to the physiologists, and who stated that they were employed by the police to collect stray dogs. I added that I regretted having been the involuntary cause of the pain which the misfortune of his dog had caused him, that the animal would not die of it, and that there was only one thing to do, namely, to let me take back my silver cannula and for him to keep the dog. These last words at once made the commissioner change his manner of speaking, and completely appeased his wife and daughter. I removed my instrument, and on leaving promised to call again. And, indeed, I visited the Rue du Jardinet several times. In a few days the dog was completely cured, I became a friend of the commissioner, and could henceforward count on his protection. Indeed this led me to establish my laboratory within his district; and for some years, until, in fact, I was appointed deputy to Magendie at the Collège de France, I was enabled to continue my private courses of experimental physiology under the licence and protection of the commissioner, whereby I was saved many disagreeable incidents."

—Claude Bernard

existed only to put out bile, an idea reminiscent of the functions assigned to the parotid gland, that of warming the ear, before Stensen's work. Bernard found that when the liver was washed out with water and was entirely free of sugar it would, if kept warm, produce sugar from some "glycogenic substance." Boiling the liver stopped this. But a combination of boiled liver and a little raw liver would once again produce sugar. So it was that Claude Bernard came to elaborate his theory of "internal secretions."

Again, from wrong premises, Claude Bernard came up undismayed with the discovery of the vasomotor nerves. He was soon back into the chorda tympani problem and discovered the difference between vaso-constrictor and vaso-dilator nerves.

In 1846 Claude Bernard quite independently found that the vagus nerve when stimulated slowed the heart—something which the brothers Weber had first communicated orally at Naples in the year 1845. Starting in 1844, Bernard set out to analyze the physiological action of the drug curare, first brought back from the New World by Sir Walter Raleigh in 1595. It was shown that the drug was harmless when swallowed because it does not diffuse into the body but that it is fatal when even the smallest amount is introduced into a surface wound of the body.

Casting back for a moment to Bernard's undergraduate days, he had already observed in 1842 the peculiar colour of the blood in cases of carbon monoxide poisoning which he had seen. By 1855 he had time to proceed with fundamental work on the problem and published on it in 1857. In the course of his work he had to develop a method for measuring the available oxygen in blood samples and was not long in reaching the conclusion that oxygen and the iron of the red corpuscles are intimately related in respiratory functions.

In 1868 Claude Bernard relinquished his chair at the Sorbonne to his pupil, Paul Bert, and moved to fine laboratories built for him at the museum of natural history by Napoleon III. He was made a senator in 1869. He was admitted to the Academie Francaise and took Flourens' seat there. Such great figures as Renan, Pasteur and Gambetta were numbered among his friends. In 1877, in the last year of his life, he returned to his two earlier themes, the gastric juice and the glycogenic function of the liver.

It should be recorded that Claude Bernard's wife and two daughters left him and turned against him, becoming anti-vivisectionists. Bernard was given a state funeral at the urging of Gambetta. His successor in L'Academie Francaise was none other than his friend Renan. The Collège de France erected a bronze statue to him in 1886, as did the faculty of medicine and science in Lyons in 1894.

It is hard to imagine a case in which the earliest interests of a medical undergraduate formed so consistently the theme of his future life's work.

Ivan Pavlov (1849-1936)

"This is in truth an amazing fact—that a recently graduated science student, who had not yet finished his medical course, became the director of scientific investigations in the most famous clinic of internal diseases in Russia." Thus does Pavlov's biographer, Boris Babkin, introduce one of the most influential student investigators of all time.

Ivan Pavlov was born in 1849, as was William Osler. At the age of twelve the "liberation of the serfs" made a great impression on him. He was educated in a church school at Ryasan and its library became one of his chief haunts. As a boy Pavlov had read a translation of G. H. Lewes' *Practical Physiology*, which was followed by I. M. Sechenov's *Reflexes of the Brain.* These two volumes he kept beside him in his library for the rest of his life. Sechenov had been greatly influenced by Darwin's *Origin of Species* which appeared just as he was graduating in medicine in Vienna.

Pavlov was attracted to medicine because of the exact methods which were just beginning to be applied in research. Sechenov's work on the organs of sense undoubtedly influenced his decision. It was the professor of physiology in the general course, Ilya Cyon, who first suggested a problem to Pavlov, and as a pre-medical student he carried on a time-consuming research on the nerves of the pancreas. For this he received a gold medal at the time of completing his pre-medical studies.

On commencing his medical student life Pavlov became an assistant in the physiological laboratory of the Veterinary Institute of the Medico-Chirurgical Academy and it was there that he did his first work on the role of nervous influences in the circulation of the blood and on the physiology of digestion.

During the summer vacation in 1877 he had the good fortune to work in the laboratory of Professor Heidenhain in Breslau, and as a result published in 1878 a paper on the effect of tying off the ducts of the pancreas in rabbits. Before he graduated, in December 1879, he published a remarkable paper on his own method of making a permanent pancreatic fistula. This method allowed him to collect the digestive juices in an active, healthy animal. This was but one of the results of the "animal clinic" which the young Pavlov set up, where the operating theatre and after-care were organized as if for human surgery. It is little wonder, then, that the distinguished clinician Botkin asked the undergraduate Pavlov to direct his research laboratory for him.

After graduation Pavlov was able to travel for two years, thanks to a fellowship. He worked in Carl Ludwig's laboratory and, for a time, in Heidenhain's laboratory again. He returned to Russia to find a new Institute of Experimental Medicine ready, and he plunged into further researches on digestion. He was given a Chair at the Military Medical Academy which he continued to hold for thirty-four years. Thus in Harvard and St. Petersburg the influence of Carl Ludwig's pupils was to be dominant for several generations of medical students. Almost contemporaneously with Cannon, Pavlov began to report on psychical factors influencing digestion in animals. In the old log buildings in the village of Koltusky Pavlov labored, despite war and revolution, and was eventually installed in beautiful quarters in the neighboring settlement of Pavlovo. There physiologists from all the world came to see him and to admire his unrivalled facilities for the care of experimental animals.

Pavlov is best known for his work on conditioned reflexes, first in association with the gastro-intestinal tract and later in the sphere of psychiatric problems. He had great faith in the explicability of human behavior as the following quotation suggests: "The time will come, even if it be remote, when mathematical analysis, based on natural scientific analysis, will embrace in its magnificent formulae all these equilibria, including finally life itself."

The current declamatory state of Russian physiology, of an official caste, does violence to Pavlov's life-long scientific activity and should not be allowed, in our minds at least, to obscure the virile life of a great discoverer. His pupils inside and outside Russia are carrying on his tradition of hard work. Pavlov's "will" had this to say to students:

"From the very beginning of your work train yourself to strict consistency in the acquirement of knowledge. . . .

"Learn the ABC of science before you attempt to scale its peaks. . . .

"Learn to do the heavy work that science involves. Study, compare, accumulate facts. . . . Without facts, your theories are labor in vain.

"Do not turn yourself into a museum custodian of facts. Try to penetrate into the secret of their origin.

"Never think that you already know everything.

"Do not allow pride to take possession of you.

"Remember that science demands a man's whole life."

Pavlov died in his eighty-fifth year, still at work in his laboratory. He was probably the best-known figure in science in post-revolutionary Russia.

Walter Bradford Cannon (1871-1945)

We swallow a great deal of food in the course of our lives in a rather automatic way—taking the process wholly for granted. In 1896 a medical student at Harvard University was puzzling over the mechanism of swallowing when he overheard a conversation in a tram, to the effect that a machine had been invented in Germany for looking right through a person.

The student, Walter Cannon, lost no time in getting to the door of his professor of physiology in the Medical School, Henry Bowditch, with a request that he be allowed to try out these new x-rays in a study of swallowing.* He had come to the right

* Visualization of the outlines of the human stomach by x-rays was pioneered in America by J. C. Hemmeter (1864-1931) in the spring of 1896 in the physics laboratory of the State Normal School, Baltimore, Maryland.

man—for Bowditch had studied in Germany under the famous Carl Ludwig who had encouraged generations of undergraduates in research projects.

With a primitive x-ray machine Cannon began his studies, knowing nothing of the dangerous radiation burns he was likely to develop in the process. He was so fearful of the sparks shot off by the machine that he shielded his body with a large sheet of lead which was at hand, thus minimizing the frightful effects which many of the early workers elsewhere suffered.

He began on December 6, 1896, by watching pearl buttons pass down the oesophagus of a dog. Twenty days afterward he was asked to demonstrate the process in a goose, before the annual meeting of the American Physiological Society. The demonstration of the orderly and rhythmic contractions of the muscular walls of the oesophagus was of great interest, since the prevailing theory was that air taken into the mouth was in some way compressed, thereby driving the food down into the stomach.

Again it was an instance where, as Pasteur said, fortune favors the prepared mind. Cannon as a pre-medical student had come under the influence of C. B. Davenport in Harvard College and had begun investigative work there in a small way on determining the influence of light on the direction and rate of movement of organisms. On entering medical school he depended for his financial support on assisting with a class in comparative anatomy at Radcliffe College nearby, and in his final year of medicine conducted this course single-handed.

We may sometimes wonder if there is really any use in searching out bright students in rural areas and in seeing that they get to University. As this chapter will show, the need to do just this is amply proven.

Walter Cannon came of French Canadian stock on his mother's side. His great-grandfather, Jacques de Noyon, escaped in the Indian massacres at Deerfield, Massachusetts, in 1704 and with his bride, Abigail Stebbins, settled on the south bank of the St. Lawrence River near Montreal, the shore which furnished medicine with another man of gastro-intestinal fame—Alexis St. Martin, the subject of William Beaumont's classical investigations on the stomach.

One of de Noyon's granddaughters, Sarah Wilma Denis (as the name became contracted) migrated to Wisconsin, settling as a teacher at Prairie du Chien. Here she married Colbert Cannon, a descendant of Samuel Carnahan (later Cannon) of Boston. Laura Cochran Cannon had walked beside her husband Samuel's covered wagon from Massachusetts to Ohio, as her great-grandson loved to tell his medical class.

To Colbert and Sarah Cannon was born Walter Bradford, in October 1871, in Prairie du Chien, which was the site of William Beaumont's second series of observations on the ever-absconding Alexis St. Martin.

Raised in St. Paul, Walter Cannon was encouraged in the use of tools by his father. One is reminded of Harvey Cushing's boyhood and of the high opinion he held of learning to use tools early in life. He said it forced one to learn to make decisions and to get on with the job.

Cannon's biological interests became apparent in high school and he was greatly influenced, as was his entire generation, by the writings of Thomas Huxley. Cannon collided with a narrow-minded family parson over such matters and withdrew from the church.

He won a freshman scholarship to Harvard, and with $180 from his family set out upon his career, being fully self-supporting from that day on. At Harvard College, as he has related in his most interesting autobiography—*The Way of an Investigator*—Cannon was, at first, at a loss to know what notes he should take at lectures. A classmate with more beef than brains advised him to take down nothing until the professor began to shout—and then to write that down verbatim!

Graduating with his B.A. degree *summa cum laude* in 1896 Cannon completed his M.A. degree and his first year of medicine together in 1897. The philosopher William James dissuaded Cannon from his one-time desire to read philosophy saying, "Don't do it, you will be filling your belly with east wind."

To return to Cannon's work as a medical student we find him perfecting a gruel of bismuth sub-nitrate which could be swallowed easily by animals in association with their normal food. His advances were communicated to the American Physiological Society, and by the time of his graduation in 1900 he was an authority on the motion of the food through the gut. (Rieder's oft-quoted paper in the German literature on the "bismuth meal" was published five years later.) There is recorded one significant exchange between Cannon, as an undergraduate, and one of the laboratory dieners or preparators. Cannon once entered the laboratory at an hour when there was no prescribed class exercise and was rudely told that no student was allowed therein. Six years later Cannon, as Bowditch's successor in the Chair of Physiology, had a chance to change this—and change it he did. There is nothing so discordant in an institution dedicated to the pursuit of knowledge as the display of usurped authority by non-teaching staff which one still finds in medical schools occasionally. The educational process, as the term implies, is "to lead out," but we are all painfully aware of how often students—the *raison d'être* of medical schools—are considered to be recurrent nuisances by departments exhibiting all the symptoms of decerebrate rigidity. Some day it will dawn on us as medical educators that it is not *our* time which is to be arranged but the *student's* time.

Cannon was "a student's professor" and his election in 1906 to Bowditch's Chair an occasion for mutual satisfaction. Bowditch had held it for thirty-five years; Cannon was to hold it for thirty-six, so that for a total of seventy-one years the benign spirit of Carl Ludwig, and his interest in student investigators, was to brood over the physiological laboratory at Harvard. Dr. Joseph Aub has recounted the fact that in his class alone, six men in their first year fell so completely under Cannon's spell that they completed investigations worthy of publication while still undergraduates. At about the same time Cannon's friend Sir Arthur Hurst was being assisted by four London medical students in an x-ray survey of the intestinal tract in normal humans. They joined him in the authorship of a paper which resulted, and which was published in Guy's Hospital Reports. All four students later distinguished themselves in separate medical specialities.

In order to help his students find their feet Cannon wrote for them an exemplary laboratory manual. His lectures always contained stimulating questions or suggestions for future investigation, and many fell on receptive ears. Since the year of Cannon's birth —1871—when the first physiological laboratory in the country was organized by Bowditch, as George Higginson Professor at Harvard, fresh ideas have been welcomed and new minds stimulated in this famous School, to the great benefit of the American people.

By the year 1912 Cannon had completed his remarkable work on the production of adrenalin in the bloodstream by such stresses as pain, low blood sugar and cold, on the rhythmic movements of the walls of the digestive tract, and on the muscle in the gut and its intrinsic and extrinsic nerve supply. He had probed the origin of "hunger pains" and surmised the psychic forces which played upon the motions and secretions of the stomach. In this connection Walter Meek has drawn attention to Michael Foster's words concerning the great physiological investigator, Claude Bernard: "The chiefest sign of genius in inquiry . . . to leave the road at the right turning and to follow a bye-path which brought him to a great result."

Cannon's turning came when one of his experimental cats became angered with him—as some cats do with experimenters occasionally—and all gastro-intestinal movements stopped, as demonstrated by x-rays. Cannon set out to find out "why," and spent his next twenty years on this phenomenon. As a result the world now knows a great deal more than it did about the emotional origin of some of its digestive upsets. Our literature was greatly enriched by the appearance in 1915 of Cannon's book, *Bodily Changes in Pain, Hunger, Fear and Rage*, and in 1932 of *The Wisdom of the Body*. He came to regard the medulla of the adrenal gland as part of the nervous system, as first suggested by a graduate student at Cambridge University, T. R. Elliott. In these "golden years" Cannon displayed the spirit of Carl Ludwig and of Purkinje, in having many of his own discoveries published by the students around him.

As an internationalist in science Cannon was saddened by the First World War. He was not long in joining the British workers under William Bayliss, however, at the laboratory for surgical research set up at Dijon.* They looked for possible "toxic factors"

* Cannon was a member of the 'Harvard Unit' which went to France long before the United States entered the war. He worked with Cuthbert Wallace at a Casualty Clearing Station and later joined the research group in London which included Bayliss, A. N. Richards and H. H. Dale.

in traumatic shock, and eventually Cannon described the condition as "toxic exemia," a view not far removed from that widely held today. For his services he was made a Commander of the Bath by King George V, and was awarded the Distinguished Service Medal by the American Government. It will be recalled that Cannon and Bayliss suggested the use of a gum acacia solution intravenously to combat shock, much as we use plasma today.

It is little wonder that in 1940 the National Research Council in Washington called Cannon to be Chairman of its Committee on Shock and Transfusion, to see if preserved blood could be made available for front line use.

Between the wars Cannon served as Exchange Professor in Paris, in 1929, and in Peiping in 1935. He visited Russia at the time of the International Physiological Congress in 1936 and formed a great affection for the Russian people.

No man of science in modern times has received so many honorary degrees, medals, and been called to so many lectureships, and yet remained so unaffected, so painstaking in his work. Cannon was very partial to the needs of the dispossessed in Spain and China. He travelled widely abroad, but also knew his homeland intimately. With his inspiring wife and five children and an indestructible Ford car he went annually to the mountains of the West for years. One of these in Glacier Park was called Mt. Cannon in his honor.

Professor Cannon died in 1945 of a white blood cell disease which first became evident in 1929. He typifies the best in American education and medicine. He was the twentieth century's Claude Bernard. His influence has been unique for no one has so fired the imagination of medical students with a belief in their worth as investigators. His pupils from almost every country in the world have taken back with them something of this spirit. As Robert Morison said in a memorial tribute: "More enduring is the feeling he left in all of us that it is possible for men throughout the world to live and work together for the common good." Generations which could not have known him will long enjoy his candid and intriguing autobiography.

PLATE 5

(a) De Graaf's illustration in his 90-page account of his student work on the pancreatic juice. From: Stirling, W.: *Some Apostles of Physiology*, London, 1902.

(b) Stensen's drawing of his undergraduate discovery (1661) of the duct of the parotid gland. From: Stirling, W.: *Some Apostles of Physiology*, London, 1902.

(c) Claude Bernard at the age of forty-three. Courtesy of the National Library of Medicine, Washington.

(d) Ivan Pavlov, 80, and Walter B. Cannon, 57, photographed at the International Physiological Congress in Boston, 1929. Courtesy of Professor Eugene Landis.

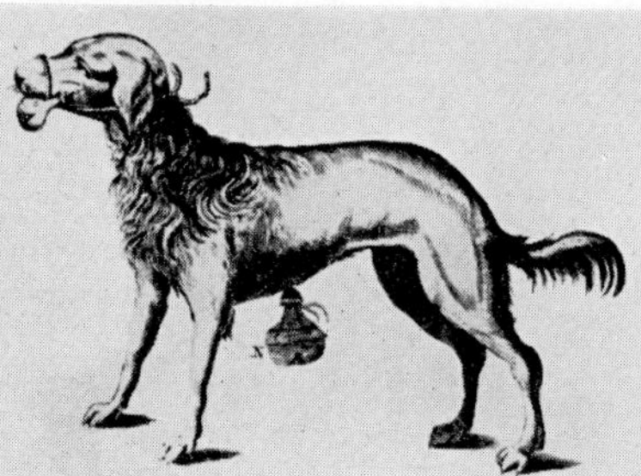

DOG WITH A PAROTID AND A PANCREATIC FISTULA, SHOWING VESSELS (A,A) FOR COLLECTING THE SALIVA AND PANCREATIC JUICE RESPECTIVELY. IT IS TAKEN FROM THE ORIGINAL FIGURE BY DE GRAAF.

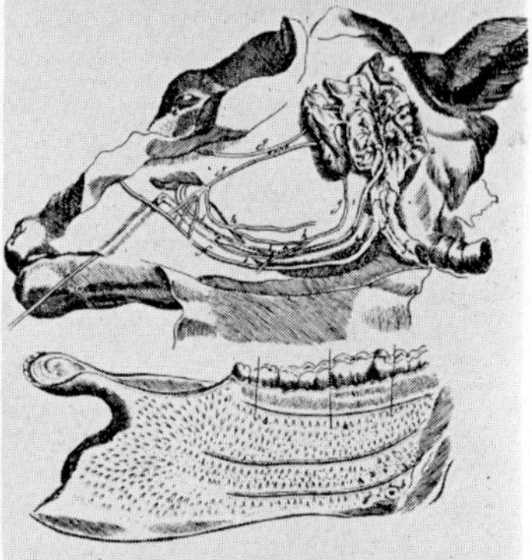

STENO'S ORIGINAL FIGURE OF THE PAROTID DUCT AND LABIAL GLANDS OF THE MOUTH OF A CALF.

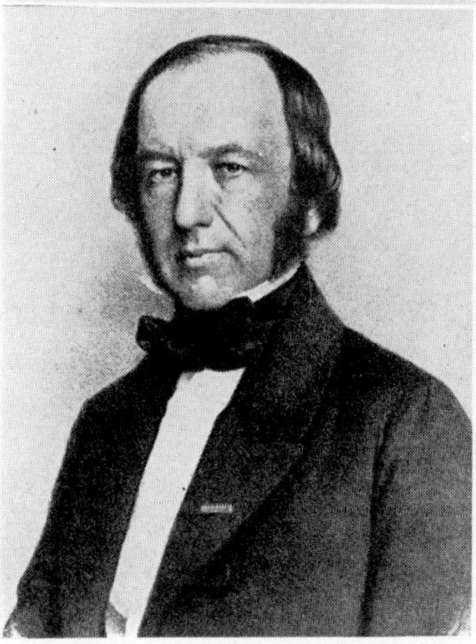

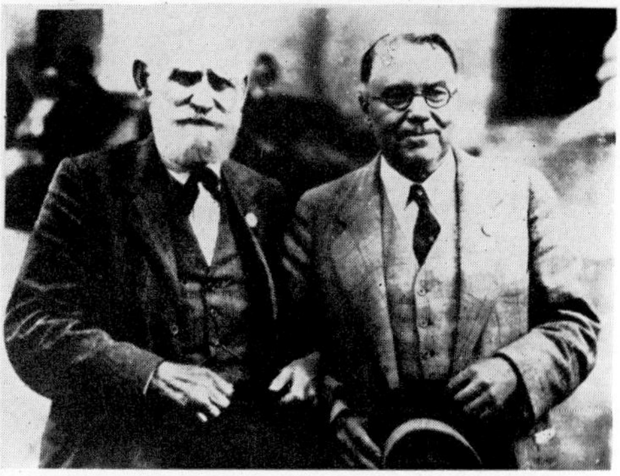

←

Chapter VII

Endocrines

THE SECOND HALF of the nineteenth century saw the unfolding of an entirely new field of medicine. While infectious diseases dominated men's minds, as well they might after the Crimean War revelations, and while aniline dyes and Darwin's views and Virchow's "cellular pathology" gained a foothold, the science of endocrinology was born. The thought that "inwardly secreting" glands existed, which produced often quite distant effects through the blood stream, was fathered by Claude Bernard in his work on the glucose role of the liver, and by Addison, in his description of the symptoms of disease of the adrenal glands. True, Bordeu had advanced such a philosophy a century earlier in France, but he had no experimental work to back it up. His clinical speculations, however, were shrewd and have a modern ring. The thyroid gland was shown by Moritz Schiff to be essential for life, and Friedleben embarked on his studies on the role of the thymus.

Paul Langerhans (1847-1888)

This is the setting in which Paul Langerhans found himself as a medical student in 1867 when he began an investigation into the microscopic structure of the pancreas. Virchow had been quick to recognize unusual qualities in this student who came from a long line of doctors, and had enabled him to work in his Institute in Berlin.

Two preliminary papers came from Langerhans' pen, on the nerves of the human skin as shown by Cohnheim's gold staining method, and on the changes seen in the tactile corpuscles in the skin during central nervous system disease. We still speak of "Langerhans' granular layer" in the skin; and of "Langerhans' stellate corpuscles" or nerve terminals in the epidermis.

In the summer vacation of 1867 Langerhans began a thorough study of the cell types encountered in the pancreas. This organ was long regarded as an abdominal salivary gland of some kind. After detailing eight already known types of cells, Langerhans, in his graduation thesis (1869) embodying his student work, described a new cell which did not conform to the assumed salivary gland picture. He saw "a small irregularly polygonal structure. Its cytoplasm is brilliant and free of any granules, its nucleus distinct, round and of moderate size. . . . These cells lie together, generally in considerable numbers, diffusely scattered in the substance of the gland."

His little thirty-one page dissertation began: "There is indeed hardly another organ in which there is such glaring contrast between the brilliant results of physiological research and the complete darkness in the realm of anatomic knowledge."

Langerhans developed a Berlin blue and glycerine mixture for the retrograde injection of the pancreatic duct, and this showed up the widely ramifying collecting system. However, his newly discovered cells bore no apparent relation to the duct system. He could see the "islets" even in a fresh rabbit pancreas, so thin were the layers in it.

This inquisitive medical student concluded his thesis with the humility which comes of hard work in the laboratory, often with meagre results: "I cannot in any way put forth the conclusive results of a completed investigation. I can describe at most a few isolated observations which suggest a much more complicated structure of the pancreas than hitherto accepted. The purpose of these lines can therefore at best be to help draw greater attention to the pancreas than has hitherto been given by anatomists."

This modest man has been sympathetically memorialized by Dr. H. Morrison of Tufts Medical School, Boston, who has translated his little thesis into English. Langerhans began his career amid the medical and political lore of a family long immersed in the life of Berlin. After a year at Jena he began the study of medicine in Berlin in 1866. After graduation he continued on in Virchow's laboratory in order to work on what we now call the reticulo-endothelial system. Within a year we find him writing to Virchow about the things he was encountering in a trip to North Africa and Asia Minor—all anthropological of course, for that was one of Virchow's great interests.

While Langerhans was made a professor of pathology in Freiburg he was forced, by a bout of tuberculosis, to give it up and to retire to Madeira. Though he continued to contribute researches on the spread of the tubercle bacillus in the body, and on leprosy, he died of his disease at the age of forty-one.

It was five years later that the generous Laguesse attached Langerhans' name to "the magic islands" discovered in the pancreas, which islands soon were credited with having an internal secretory activity, in close association with capillaries and nerves. In fact Laguesse started off the series of events which led Von Mehring and Minkowski, Opie and Ssobolew, W. G. MacCallum, and finally Banting and Best into the study of the islet cells which in 1922 resulted in the development from them of life-giving "insulin."

Thus did a medical student's little dissertation start off a chain of development of inestimable value.*

Ivar Sandstrom (1852-1889)

When Santiago Ramón y Cajal visited Stockholm to receive the Nobel Prize in medicine he remarked that gray matter flourished under gray skies. This was certainly true in the case

* Jean Conrad Brunner (1653-1727) discovered the glands still known as Brunner's glands in the submucosa of the duodenum at the age of nineteen though he did not publish his work on them until fifteen years later when he became Professor of Medicine at Heidelberg. His early study was done at Strasbourg. Brunner thought of his glands as "a secondary pancreas" secreting a similar kind of substance. In fact Brunner partly removed the spleen and pancreas from dogs and found that in one dog at least, great thirst and frequent micturition, together with a ravenous appetite, ensued.

of Ivar Sandstrom, who, as a student in the pre-clinical course at Uppsala in 1877, discovered the parathyroid glands.

Today we know how important these minute structures are for the regulation of calcium metabolism in the body. Fatal muscle spasms or tetany may follow their accidental removal during thyroid operations. In 1877, however, no one knew of this connection. It took a dogged medical student three years to round out even the anatomical picture, so hard pressed was he with his prescribed studies. It was to be an erstwhile student discoverer —William G. MacCallum of malaria fame—who worked out the calcium regulating rôle of the parathyroids in 1905 at the age of thirty-one.

The thoroughness of Sandstrom's gross and microscopic observations was such that his descriptions have hardly been bettered over the intervening years. Dr. Carl M. Seipel has translated Sandstrom's account into English. With engaging simplicity this student began:

> About three years ago (1877) I found on the thyroid gland of a dog a small organ, hardly as big as a hemp seed, which was enclosed in the same connective tissue capsule as the thyroid, but could be distinguished therefrom by a lighter color. A superficial examination revealed an organ of a totally different structure from that of the thyroid, and with a very rich vascularity. . . . The existence of a hitherto unknown gland in animals that have so often been a subject of anatomical examination called for a thorough approach to the region around the thyroid gland, even in man. . . . It was exclusively with the purpose of completing the investigation, rather than with the hope of finding something new that I began a careful examination of this region. So much the greater was my astonishment therefore when in the first individual examined I found on both sides at the inferior border of the thyroid gland an organ of the size of a small pea, which, judging from its exterior, did not appear to be a lymph gland, not an accessory thyroid gland, and upon histological examination showed a rather peculiar structure. . . .

The great vascularity of this endocrine or hormone-secreting tissue had greatly impressed Sandstrom. As he prepared to show some microscopic slides of his early work to his sympathetic teacher, Professor Edward Clason, Sandstrom looked into Clason's microscope which was at that moment focussed on a section of the pituitary gland. Struck by the similarity of the glandular tissue shot through with myriad blood vessels, Sandstrom cried out in amazement: "Have you already seen the gland I was going to show you?"

We have noted that Sandstrom's description was thorough and painstaking. In fact it was too thorough for the editors of a German scientific periodical to whom it was submitted, unsuccessfully, for publication. For this reason the world knew little of the work except for Retzius' review in a German yearbook. In 1892 Gley "rediscovered" the glands, and brought Sandstrom's work before the world. Actually, Richard Owen in 1850 read a paper to the Zoological Society of London on the parathyroid glands of the Great Indian Rhinoceros which died in 1849, having been bought for 1,000 guineas in 1834! Of course, Sandstrom's microscopic work on the gland was his real contribution, which is not to decry his own independent finding of the glands in the much-dissected dog!

Sandstrom knew what he was about, and he knew his limitations. He concludes his work thus: "While working on the above description of these hitherto unrecognized organs, I have tried to go through the older as well as the newer literature in order to find out whether these glands have been previously known and then forgotten again—but unfortunately, the literature which I have had at my disposal has been too scanty and too hard of access for these studies to pretend to be complete." He then quotes Remak and Virchow, both student contributors whom we have encountered, who had more or less rudimentary descriptions of the gland but nothing as detailed as Sandstrom's material.

It is interesting to read Sandstrom's student paper for its grasp of general anatomy. He mentions, for instance, the signs and symptoms which one might expect from a tumor or swelling of the parathyroids, as judged from their proximity to the oesophagus and to the recurrent laryngeal nerve supplying the vocal cords. Again, Sandstrom looked for, but did not find, some close relation between the gland and the lymphatic vessels. He was obviously testing out its possible role as a lymph gland. The volume of work undertaken and completed by this medical student brings a feeling of fatigue to the reader. He dissected out the glands of a large variety of mammals and examined their position and minute structure in fifty humans.

The thoroughness demonstrated in this work also is to be found in Sandstrom's method of teaching histology or microscopic anatomy. His later students at Uppsala studied histology at the microscope, while he lectured to the class. They became literate in the subject by actually making the slide their textbook, there being no intermediary.

Sandstrom came of a family of public servants and scholars. In his short life of thirty-seven years he accomplished a great deal, despite recurrent mental illness. His contribution provided not only the framework for the future physiology of calcium regulation in the body but also for an understanding of some of the hazards of thyroid surgery. His work, too long unrecognized, is a tribute to all medical students who have pioneered and to the sympathetic teachers who have encouraged them.

Pierre Marie (1853-1940)

Neurologists the world over claim Pierre Marie as one of the most brilliant founders of their specialty. Why then is he included in a chapter on endocrinology?

As a medical student Marie became interested in the tremor, especially visible in the extended arms and fingers, in cases of thyroid disease in which an excess of this hormone is released into the bloodstream. His graduation thesis in 1883 first graphically presented this sign, which every medical student today searches for in doing a physical examination. Under the tutelage of the great clinician Charcot he grew up in the wards of the Salpêtrière in Paris, observing clinical abnormalities and then pursuing them to the pathological laboratory for an explanation.

It was in this manner that Marie, with Charcot, described the disease known as peroneal muscular atrophy in 1886, just three years after Marie had qualified in medicine. This work took him on an excursion into pathology, the laws of heredity, muscle diseases and electrophysiology. In the same year, Tooth, in his Cambridge M.D. thesis, described the same features of the disease, and his name is today coupled with those of Marie and Charcot in its definition.

Marie's fame as an endocrinologist rests upon his thorough description of acromegaly, that disease which Marie may have seen as he walked through the streets of Paris—the large head and the enormous extremities. As he studied these people in hospital he learned that they also had large tongues, headache and increasing visual difficulty, an intense thirst with a great outpouring of sugary urine, and with either amenorrhoea or impotence. In reviewing an autopsy performed when he was a student in 1882, Marie found that the acromegalic patient, Henri Honrot, had secreted within the pituitary fossa in the base of his skull a tumor resembling a hen's egg in size. The enlarged pituitary fossa of another case of Marie's was later described by the ever-enquiring Broca and gradually the pituitary origin of acromegaly came to be established. Finally in 1921 the patient and pioneering work of Herbert Evans and Long showed that the growth hormone found in the anterior part of the pituitary gland was definitely responsible for the production of gigantism.*

As Sir Henry Cohen has shown in his paper read to the Royal Society of Medicine in 1953, Pierre Marie's life is one of extraordinary interest—filled with triumphs of observation, generalization and fertile imagination. It is filled, alas, with sorrows, too. He was born in Paris and attended a classical school at Vauves. His father persuaded him to study law and he was actually called to the bar. However, his desire to study medicine was unabated and he turned to this calling with both enthusiasm and a broad preparation. His knowledge of foreign languages, history and art were to mark him out as an exceptional medical student, and it is little wonder that Charcot came to regard him as his most accomplished disciple.

In temperament precise and exacting—possibly as a result of the military discipline of his early schooling, and of his legal

* It might not be amiss to note here parenthetically that one of the best researches done on the posterior pituitary and its function was carried out by the late Alexander M. Fraser as a first year medical student at McGill University, Montreal, in the summer vacation of 1935. It is a matter for profound regret that following a brilliant wartime career of hazardous investigation into high altitude problems he succumbed to cancer in his early thirties.

training—Marie was nevertheless a great teacher. He was deaf to the blandishments of Paris society. He lived for his patients and his family. In turn his daughter, his wife and his son died of infections which today would have been curable. Just before the fall of Paris, Marie was operated upon for an abdominal condition by Count Thierry de Martel—the surgeon who was soon to commit suicide rather than make his life "a blank cheque," as he said, for the invading Nazis. Marie died on April 13, 1940, at the age of eighty-seven, on the Côte d'Azur which he loved so well. Endocrinology and neurology had been powerfully influenced by this one-time lawyer and student contributor.

The triumvirate of Langerhans, Sandstrom and Pierre Marie illustrates the opportunities which were exploited by a microscopist, a gross anatomist and a clinical observer, respectively. The field of endocrinology probably offers more scope than any other today for further observations by enquiring medical students.

Chapter VIII

Infection and Pathology

"The history of the discovery of the 'germ' world, the genius and painstaking ability of the early pioneers, the dangers they underwent, the difficulties they overcame, the disappointments they encountered, and the triumphs they achieved, make up a story of almost unbelievable interest.

"The path of most pioneers is a hard and thorny one and the path of these early bacteriologists was one of difficulty and constant danger. Every obstacle was placed in their way by colleagues who had neither the sense nor the intellect to see that a new world was being opened up by these despised workers in the realm of the unseen. They were derided and scorned for holding their opinions but they kept on and finally unfolded a world of previously unseen fantastic microscopic creatures whose existence had never before been dreamed of. Perhaps the only thing in their favor was the fact that there were no Home Office regulations with regard to animal experimentation."

—Arthur Bulleid

Edward Jenner (1749-1823)

THERE IS a legend that Edward Jenner, as a medical apprentice near Bristol, at the age of nineteen, grasped the significance of the age-old tale that an attack of cowpox prevented smallpox, and that his medical student life in London and his life as a practitioner in Gloucestershire revolved about this concept. It is only a legend, however, without any firm proof.

Jenner may well have decided, when a child of eight years, that something simpler was required, as a preventive of smallpox, than the "variolation" to which he was then subjected. The procedure involved the transfer of infected matter from a known case of smallpox to a person by direct inoculation, once the person to be protected had been bled, purged and starved for six weeks beforehand!

Jenner was born in 1749—an even hundred years before Osler—in a manse also. His father was the Vicar of Berkeley in the lovely county of Gloucestershire. As a boy Edward had a large collection of fossils and nests. He was a keen observer of nature, and his ability in this field was later recognized by Captain Cook whose specimens of the natural history of Australia Jenner examined and prepared in 1771. Cook invited Jenner in 1772 to accompany him on the second expedition but Jenner the medical student, by then apprenticed to John Hunter in London, decided against it. In fact his refusal of this tempting offer is responsible for Jenner's fame in the cardio-vascular field. In the same year he made his first observations on a case of angina pectoris which had been treated by Heberden. The patient had warned his physician of his painful chest symptoms and on his death John Hunter was called in to perform an examination of the heart. Jenner mentions this case of anginal distress as "the first I ever saw." His interest in heart disease never abated, though he had to maintain silence on his teacher John Hunter's condition which was clearly one of angina pectoris—"this dreadful disease." Years later Jenner wrote concerning an autopsy examination of the heart which he had performed that his "knife struck against something so hard and gritty that I well remember looking up to the ceiling conceiving that some plaster had fallen down." Jenner's paper, "Remarks on a Disease of the Heart Following Acute Rheumatism, Illustrated by Dissections" (1789), antedates all others on this important subject by twenty years.

The observant medical student became, through John Hunter's constant stimulus, a keen clinical observer upon beginning practice in Berkeley in 1773. To Jenner we owe the first clear statement of the allergic phenomenon known as "anaphylaxis," which means literally "backward protection." It refers to the hypersusceptibility of the body to a second injection of a foreign protein following upon a first after an interval of time.

The setting was this. A patient, Mary Barge, had suffered from smallpox some time previous to 1791. In that year Jenner injected into her some living smallpox virus to determine how much resistance she had built up as a result of her previous infection. Of the dramatic skin reaction which followed, Jenner wrote: "It is remarkable that variolous matter when the system is disposed to reject it should excite inflammation . . . more speedily than when it produces the smallpox. . . . It seems as if a change, which endures through life, had been produced in the action or disposition to action, in the vessels of the skin. . . . Whether this change has been effected by the smallpox or the cowpox the disposition to sudden cuticular inflammation is the same on the application of variolous matter."

Jenner had both brains and time to use them. He reflected on the most amazing things, always in search of unifying general principles. He thought that there was "a sympathy between the constitution and the skin, in all probability through the brain and nervous system"—long before the embryologist Robert Remak showed, in 1845, that the nervous system is derived from the primitive skin or ectoderm.

Writing in the publication known as *The Artist* in 1807, Jenner discussed "Classes of the Human Powers of Intellect"—and listed, 1: The Idiot—"the mere vegetative being;" 2: The Dolt—"the weak, silly, poor creature;" 3: Mediocrity—"the large mass of mankind;" 4: Mental Perfection—"From this point Intellect again diverges;" 5: Eccentricity—"I have in this class a very numerous acquaintance;" 6: Insanity—"the most affecting of all conditions;" illustrated from the life of William Cowper, whose verses are quoted; 7: The Maniac—"the wreck of mental faculties."

The many-sided nature of Jenner is beautifully portrayed by his biobibliographer, W. R. LeFanu (1951). As a poet Jenner was definitely gifted. He was interested in aeronautics and in 1783, the year in which Montgolfier's balloon ascended to one thousand feet in France, Jenner built a balloon in the great hall of Berkeley Castle, and after filling it with hydrogen watched it rise over the Vale. It was retrieved several miles away and recharged for another ascent.

In 1796—twenty-three years after completing his training at St. George's Hospital, London, Jenner vaccinated his first case. James Phipps, a boy of eight years, was protected by vaccination on May 14, 1796 from a pustule on the arm of Sarah Nelmes, a dairy maid with cowpox, against smallpox injected on July 1, 1796. Jenner wrote:

> I selected a healthy boy (James Phipps) about eight years old, for the purpose of inoculation for the cow-pox. The matter was taken from a sore on the hand of a dairy maid (Sarah Nelmes) who was infected by her master's cows, and it was inserted, on the 14th day of May, 1796, into the arm of the boy by means of two superficial incisions, barely penetrating the cutis, each about half an inch long.
>
> On the seventh day he complained of uneasiness in the axilla and on the ninth he became a little chilly, lost his apetite, and had a slight headache. During the whole of this day he was perceptibly indisposed, and spent the night with some degree of restlessness, but on the day following he was perfectly well. . . . In order to ascertain whether the boy, after feeling so slight an affection of the system from the cow-pox virus, was secure from contagion of the smallpox, he was inoculated on the 1st of July following with variolous matter, immediately taken from a pustule. Several slight punctures and incisions were made on both his arms, and the matter was carefully inserted, but no disease followed. . . . Several months afterward he was again inoculated with variolous matter, but no sensible effect was produced on the condition.

Jenner sought to interest physician friends on a visit to London and left a little of the cow-pox virus with the surgeon, Mr. Cline, at St. Thomas' Hospital. Cline became convinced of the great protective value of the vaccine and promised Jenner an income of £10,000 per year if he would come to London. Jenner's famous reply was this:

> Shall I, who even in the morning of my days sought the lowly and sequestered paths of life, the valley, and not the mountain;

shall I now my evening is fast approaching, hold myself up as an object for fortune and for fame? Admitting it as a certainty that I obtain both, what stock should I add to my little fund of happiness? My fortune, with what flows in from my profession, is sufficient to gratify my wishes; indeed, so limited is my ambition, and that of my nearest connexions, that were I precluded from further practice, I should be enabled to obtain all I want. And as for fame, what is it? a gilded butt, forever pierced with the arrows of malignancy.

Oxford University honoured itself by making Jenner a Doctor of Physic fifteen years after the "Inquiry" was published. The College of Physicians in London refused to admit him except by examination. But less rigid minds from all corners of the world sought to learn from Jenner and to bless him. Thomas Jefferson, and Benjamin Waterhouse, "the American Jenner," corresponded with him, and the "Five Nations" of North American Indians sent him effusive thanks for his help in devising a plan for their vaccination. They wrote: "We shall not fail to teach our children to speak the name of Jenner and to thank the Great Spirit for bestowing on him so much wisdom and benevolence." Jenner's life demonstrates the approach of the investigator, best epitomized in the memorable advice of his teacher John Hunter, "But why think, why not try the experiment?"

TUBERCULOSIS

René Theophile Hyacinth Laennec (1781-1826)

The mention of the name Laennec brings at once to mind the word "auscultation"—the art of listening through the stethoscope—the invention of Laennec. Little do we realize, as we think of the great clinical triumphs of this French physician, that his undergraduate publications were works of a high order also.

He was born on February 17, 1781 at Quimper in Western Brittany, in a granite house on the quay overlooking the junction of the Steir and the Odet Rivers. His ancestors were magistrates, sailors and poets of Celtic stock. At an early age Laennec's mother died in childbirth, leaving her husband with three small children. Laennec's uncle, who was a priest, educated the two boys of the family, until he was forced to flee to England after the clergy were proscribed. He died in Southampton of tuberculosis, March 18, 1800.

Thereupon René Laennec who was the eldest of the family journeyed with the younger brother to Nantes to join another uncle, Guillaume, who was a physician, and Rector of the University of Nantes at the age of forty. He had been a pupil of John Hunter in England.

During the unsettled revolutionary period in France, the steadying influence of Uncle Guillaume was a very important factor in Laennec's development. A guillotine set up before his uncle's house at Nantes took the lives of 3,000 citizens before the bloodshed was brought to a halt in that northwest corner of France. It is hard to conceive in these circumstances that Laennec started writing poetry at the age of eleven. In September, 1795 he entered the School of Medicine, University of Nantes, conducted in the Hotel Dieu. He was then just fourteen years old. It was not long before he was enrolled as a military surgeon, third class. Even at this age he was a confirmed naturalist, a trait which he shared with others discussed in this book, such as William Osler, Edward Jenner, Richard Bright and Frederick Gowland Hopkins. He was a good Greek scholar and he loved to play the flute. Unfortunately, his early life was dogged by constant lack of funds. It is recorded that on one occasion he walked all the way from Nantes to Quimper and back in a fruitless effort to get money from his father to help with his studies. When René's father and step-mother tried to keep him in Quimper in order to enter into the business of the family, Uncle Guillaume wrote them: "For God's sake let him come back to me as I sent him to you, good, gentle and studious; let him pursue in peace a course of study which is good for his health, sufficient for his fortune and honourable for his reputation." Finally in 1801, he was able to procure a legal order on his father which bound him to assist the son to continue his medical undergraduate work in Paris.

Entering L'École de Médicine in Paris in May of the same year, Laennec took his instruction at La Charité under Corvisart, the translator of Auenbrugger's work on percussion. Laennec wrote voluminous notes on all that he saw and heard. In his three years at La Charité as an undergraduate he wrote meticulous case-histories on four hundred patients, which fact might well be brought to the attention of present day undergraduates at the beginning of each new academic year. Though Laennec knew German and English he continued to study his Greek and it is little wonder that his graduation thesis presented in 1804 concerned Hippocrates. Few students today read Hippocrates and fewer still read him in Greek.

In his thesis, "Propositions on the Teaching of Hippocrates Relative to Medicine," Laennec wrote:

> The only method by which one can acquire solid knowledge in medicine depends on avoiding the adoption of any principle which is not proven by many individual facts; by studying with care the character and course of diseases and by treating them according to the indications drawn from the observations of that which has succeeded in like cases. This is the method which Hippocrates asserts to have been known long before him, which he presents as the only way by which one may make real discoveries.

Laennec's letters to his father during his final year in medical school showed the development of his work on the arachnoid or "spidery" membrane which covers the brain, and on the synovial membranes which line the joints of the extremities.

Almost from his first day in Medicine in Paris Laennec was interested in investigation. In his first year he was chosen a member of the Society of Medical Instruction at which students presented case histories and pathological reports. He joined Dupuytren in working on morbid anatomy and became an enthusiastic disciple of Bichat who died the following year, aged thirty-one. In 1802, at the age of twenty-one, Laennec published his first paper on a case of mitral disease. Two months later he published "a fine piece of original work," as Sir William Hale-White has described it, on the inflammation of the peritoneum. Some of the terms which Laennec introduced in this paper are still in use today. He was soon recognized by his teachers as something new on the horizon. He wrote on venereal disease, suicide, amenorrhoea, and on the lining of the cerebral ventricles. In 1803 he announced his discovery of the subdeltoid bursa and soon produced a paper on "the tunics which envelope certain viscera," in which he showed clearly that Glisson's capsule around the liver was not, as some said, muscular in nature. In 1804 he read his paper on hydatids to the Society of the Medical School and contrary to the current dogma showed that the cysts were due to parasites. During this year also he was able to complete part of a book, "Traité sur l'anatomie pathologique," which remained in manuscript form until edited by Cornil eighty years later.

Laennec finished his undergraduate career by being made an editor of the *Journal of Medicine, Surgery and Pharmacy*, to which he had already contributed so much in the way of new pathological concepts. In contrast to his great success in his studies, his financial worries became worse, and he wrote to his father that for lack of decent clothes he would probably have to postpone his graduation examinations.

Laennec began practice rather inauspiciously, showing on his account books for the first year only 150 francs, and for the second year 400 francs. But as Osler remarks, "He had much capital in his brainpan." One wonders how much was expected of a recent graduate of the year 1804. Laennec's practical examination in surgery had involved the amputation of the humerus at the shoulder joint! His first assistant on this occasion, however, was the great surgeon Dupuytren, so we may assume that he could not have gone far wrong.

Laennec was catapulted to fame by his invention of the stethoscope in 1817. For centuries children had been playing a game of tapping on the ends of logs or pipes while others listened to the transmitted sound. It remained for Laennec with his outstanding preparation in pathological anatomy, as we have seen, to employ this elementary principle of "auscultation" in the diagnosis of pulmonary and cardiac disease in the living patient. Only two years after his invention of the stethoscope he published the work which made him famous at once throughout the world. With his own lathe he made stethoscopes for those who sought to verify statements in his book! Seven years later he published a second edition which was enlarged to include the underlying pathology, the diagnosis, and the method of treatment of each disease discussed in a systematic manner. For the first time, and

"In 1816, I was consulted by a young woman labouring under general symptoms of diseased heart, and in whose case percussion and the application of the hand were of little avail on account of the great degree of fatness. The other method just mentioned (ear to chest method of Hippocrates) being rendered inadmissible by the age and sex of the patient, I happened to recollect a simple and well-known fact in acoustics, and fancied at the same time, that it might be turned to some use on the present occasion. The fact I allude to is the augmented impression of sound when conveyed through certain solid bodies, as when we hear the scratch of a pin at one end of a piece of wood, in applying our ear to the other. Immediately, on this suggestion, I rolled a quire of paper into a sort of cylinder and applied one end of it to the region of the heart and the other to my ear, and was not a little surprised and pleased, to find that I could thereby perceive the action of the heart in a manner much more clear and distinct than I had ever been able to do by the immediate application of the ear. From this moment I imagined that the circumstance might furnish means of enabling us to ascertain the character, not only of the action of the heart, but of every species of sound produced by motion of all the thoracic viscera."

(From "Auscultation Médiate" by R. T. H. Laennec. 1819.
Forbes translation.)

in a manner never equalled since, Laennec put the diagnosis of diseases of the lungs and of the heart and, for that matter, all intrathoracic diseases, on a sound basis through his masterly correlation of the physical signs which he listed with the pathological processes at work.

The fact is that the very terms which we use today were introduced by this restless and thorough investigator. Osler bade his students read Laennec in the original on the diagnosis of pneumonia. Again we see Laennec's student preparation coming out as he discusses in his great text of 1826 the problems of peritonitis, cirrhosis of the liver (which today bears his name), cancer of the lung, pneumothorax, tuberculosis, pleurisy, emphysema and bronchiectasis. The simplicity and directness of his writings are illustrated in the following passage taken from Forbes' translation, *Pulmonary Respiration.*

> "On applying the cylinder to the breast of a healthy person, we hear, during inspiration and expiration, a slight but distinct murmur, answering to the entrance of the air into, and its expulsion from the air cells of the lung. This murmur may be compared to that produced by a pair of bellows whose valve makes no noise, or, still better, to that emitted by a person in a deep and placid sleep who makes now and then a profound inspiration. The moist crepitous rattle has evidently its site in the substance of the lungs. It resembles the sound produced by the crepitation of salts in a vessel exposed to a gentle heat or that produced by blowing into a dried bladder, or it is still more like that emitted by the healthy lungs when distended by air and compressed in the hand—only stronger. Besides the sound of crepitation, a sensation of humidity in the part is clearly conveyed . . . it is the pathognomonic sign of the first stage of peripneumony, disappearing on the supervention of hepatization and reappearing with the resolution of the inflammation."

The publication of Laennec's great "Traité de l'auscultation médiate" found him in very poor health and he rested for two years near his home in Quimper, at a delightful seacoast spot "Kerlouarnec"—literally "The place of the foxes." His practice had been overwhelming him, so that he sought on his return to Paris to concentrate on his teaching as Professor of Medicine at the Collège de France.

In 1824 Laennec married Madame Guichard-Gueguen. He was made a Knight of the Legion of Honour as his fame increased. The second edition of his book exhausted him and again, in 1826, he returned to Kerlouarnec where he died of tuberculosis at the age of forty-five. Thus did the meteoric inventor of the stethoscope wear himself out. His early uphill struggles may have cost him his health, but they never modified his great charm and sense of humour. Laennec died in 1826 but he remains one of the best-known and certainly the best-loved discoverers and teachers of all time.

The first English book (1825) on the value and use of Laennec's stethoscope was written by a twenty-one year old medical student at Edinburgh, William Stokes (1804-1878). It was entitled: "An introduction to the use of the stethoscope; with its application to the diagnosis in disease of the thoracic viscera; including the pathology of these various affections." For this 226-page volume, William Stokes received the sum of £70.

In Dublin, three years later, Stokes was publishing two lectures which foreshadowed his great work (1837) on *Diseases of the Chest*. The account of Stokes-Adams disease—slow pulse with fainting attacks—was published when Stokes was 42, and the paper on Cheyne-Stokes respiration—cyclic increase and decrease in respiratory rate—appeared in 1854.

Stokes, with his colleague Graves, made Dublin a mecca for medical men of the last century. He succeeded his father as Regius Professor of Medicine there at the age of 38, and served thus for 36 years.

As Laennec was leaving the stage a young American, James Jackson, Jr., of Boston, was entering Harvard University. He was to follow in the French clinical tradition and to gain fame in a too-short life of twenty-four years. His father, James Jackson (1777-1868), a dresser of Sir Astley Cooper, and first physician to the Massachusetts General Hospital, was well known for his early writing on the mental symptoms of alcoholic neuritis resulting from drinking "ardent spirits," and on typhoid fever. His name will live in medical literature, however, as the author of *A Memoir of James Jackson, Jr.* (1835) and *Letters to a Young*

Physician (1855). Of the *Memoir* Osler wrote that it should be "put in the way of" all medical students; "few biographies will do them more good."

James Jackson, Jr. (1810-1834) entered Harvard Medical Faculty after taking his B.A. degree in 1828. As a second year student in the Massachusetts General Hospital he won distinction as one of the Boylston essay prize winners. In the spring of 1831 he sought the wards of the great Paris teacher Pierre Charles Alexandre Louis (1787-1872), as did the sons of such other Boston medical men as John Collins Warren of ether fame, and Nathaniel Bowditch the patron saint of navigators. Louis took a truly fatherly interest in this gifted young American, and granted him (and Oliver Wendell Holmes) free access to his wards at the Charité Hospital, an honour rarely bestowed upon students.

Jackson worked incessantly under his inspiring master, and in the midst of a frightful epidemic of cholera which beset Paris in 1832, he found time to send a 212-page memoir back to Boston on the outbreak! He belonged to the "Societé Médicale d'Observation de Paris," of which Louis was president. Attendance at its weekly meeting was compulsory for those few elected to membership, which included Marshall Hall, Chomel, Andral, Bowditch and O. W. Holmes. In 1833, before this society, the ever-observant Jackson read a paper in which there is reported for the first time the prolonged expiratory sound to be heard in the chests of early cases of tuberculosis. Jackson's studies on emphysema, while still an undergraduate, marked him as one with a great future.

Louis wrote most touching letters to Jackson's father in Boston, beseeching him to leave his son another year in Paris that he might carry further his interests in clinical pathology. However, in the latter part of 1833 Jackson, Jr. made his way home to Boston to prepare for his examinations for the Doctorate in medicine. He contracted dysentery and died March 27, 1834.

The field of tuberculosis was to attract another student contributor, James Blake (1815-1893), whose early chemical work, antedating the periodic table, is reviewed in another chapter of this book (p. 79). Blake's activities in the care of tuberculous patients were centred in California, where in 1860 he published a report of the success of his open-air rest treatment of such cases and later developed a sanitarium near Mount St. Helena, California.

Lastly, in point of time, we come to Robert Koch (1843-1910), the country doctor whose contributions to our knowledge of tuberculosis were monumental. One of thirteen children, he was born in Hanover in 1843, and developed into a keen athlete, a boy interested in music and in natural history as provided in the surrounding countryside by botanizing, and by mineralizing with his father, a mining engineer of note.

Koch's medical training began at the age of nineteen, at the University of Göttingen under such active and renowned scientists as Krause in pathology, Meissner in physiology, Henle in anatomy and Wöhler, the first man to synthesize an organic compound from inorganic chemicals in a test tube. In 1824, at the age of 24, Wöhler had already upset current theory by showing that animals as well as plants can build up very complex molecules from simple dietary constituents. The spirit of enquiry was certainly abroad in this medical school.

While a third-year student Koch won first prize in the annual essay contest in the medical faculty, the subject in 1865 being the nerve supply to the uterus. Professor Krause was so impressed that he appointed Koch as his assistant in the Pathological Museum, and thus opened the door to a whole new world—that of the microscopic observation of diseased tissue. The lad who had learned the art of careful observation in botany and mineralogy was now to practise it in that starkly real world of human life and death. His apprenticeship in the museum was brief, but it impressed on his fertile mind the overwhelming value of method in research.

For his graduation dissertation Koch described the experimental work which he had carried on for some time under Meissner in the Physiological Institute. It was the "metabolic" era, and Koch was studying the excretion of succinic acid in animals fed upon nothing but fat and meat. He was a spirited investigator and tested meals on himself—such as eating half a pound of butter at once and then calculating his output of succinic acid. His research brought forth great praise at the time of his graduation in medicine, *cum laude*, in January 1866.

Ten years and three months later a country doctor who had been through the Franco-Prussian war and had worked, in hours wrung from his busy rural practice, at a microscope in a little cubicle in his examining room, astonished the scientific world with his claim that he had completely explained the life cycle of the deadly anthrax bacillus which plagued his farming community. He revealed his discoveries to a botanist in Breslau, Ferdinand Cohn, who lost no time in inviting him to come with his materials to demonstrate his work to the medical giants Weigert, Auerbach, Traube, and Cohnheim the distinguished pathologist.

Thus, Robert Koch, the once promising medical student, lost from sight in a rural practice, kept the flame of research burning, as Jenner, Sir James MacKenzie and Withering did, in their country callings. Koch showed that the anthrax bacillus could be cultured outside the body, generation after generation, and could yet cause the disease when injected into animals. Then came his work on the staining and photography of bacteria—methods now used daily all over the world—but applied then only in a little cubicle in a German country doctor's office, devoid of all chromium plate, innocent of personnel directors, and unbaptized by any liturgy of "foundationese."

Within two years of the first bombshell Koch was reporting on the bacterial flora of infected wounds. With all this discovered, Koch was propelled by Cohnheim to the Imperial Health Department where he soon developed the gelatin plate method of pure culturing of bacteria. This method opened a whole new vista to bacteriological researchers. Finally, in 1882, Koch demonstrated the bacillus responsible for tuberculosis. He went on to develop his "postulates" on the nature of the incriminating evidence necessary to convict a specific organism as causing a disease; he hoped that tuberculin would aid early cases of tuberculosis—a hope shared fifty years later by Sir Hugh Cairns at Oxford as he successfully attacked tuberculous meningitis.

At the University of Berlin Koch developed a laboratory

which trained the students, including Sherrington, who were to take his teachings and, more importantly, his research methods to the four corners of the world. The award of the Nobel Prize in Medicine in 1905 crowned a great career in one who brought the cure of tuberculosis immeasurably nearer because he discovered its cause.

Thus, tuberculosis was studied by an interesting group of men whose undergraduate years were filled with unanswered questions and the encouragement of good teachers. Laennec's quest for knowledge was aided by his Uncle Guillaume whose enquiring mind reflected his early training with John Hunter in London. William Stokes was caught up by the same Scottish spirit of observation that caused his classmate James Hope (1801-1841) to write his graduating thesis on "Aneurysm of the Aorta," and only six years later to present to the world his classic *Diseases of the Heart and Great Vessels.* James Jackson, Jr. drank at the fountain of the immortal Louis, a great teacher because self-taught. Blake fell under the spell of William Sharpey, a Scot teaching physiology at University College, London, who was to launch Joseph Lister, ere long, as a student researcher. Last of the group, we find the enterprising student Robert Koch surrounded by teachers with vision and great talent.

CHILD-BED FEVER

"Child-bed fever," or puerperal sepsis, is an illness whose very name still strikes terror into the heart. No scourge more sorrow-laden was ever known, and none more needless can be imagined. Two erstwhile law students, Oliver Wendell Holmes and Ignaz Semmelweis, remain the best-known crusaders against the scourge, though the youthful Charles White (1728-1813), who at the age of twenty-four was instrumental in founding the Manchester Infirmary, also reduced maternal mortality on his wards by cleanliness and by isolating infected cases.

The preparation of Holmes and Semmelweis for the rôle in which Fate eventually cast them was not some stereotyped curriculum in which "the right answers" were learned. Holmes, the Boston intellectual, and Semmelweis, the Hungarian patriot, made strange bedfellows, but their informed and fearless campaign changed history.

Holmes was born in 1809 into the liberal atmosphere of Rev. Abiel Holmes' and Sarah Wendell's family circle. On both sides of the family tree there were doctors. From his mother he inherited spirit, and from his Yale-taught father a taste for revelry which was to break out repeatedly in The Hasty Pudding Club and in other waggish pursuits at Harvard.

As a boy, O. W. Holmes was in almost daily contact with "The American Jenner"—as their neighbor Dr. Benjamin Waterhouse called himself. Holmes took up dancing and cigars at an early age and, being ready prematurely to enter Harvard, was sent to school for a year at Andover, where he developed a taste for oratory.

At the age of sixteen, and being all of 5 feet 3 inches tall, he entered Harvard College, where he became famed for his humorous verse. With his friends he produced an exact copy of the sober Harvard Triennial Catalogue, in which they gave themselves a host of honorary degrees! Rev. Abiel Holmes found it hard to squelch this exuberance since he, in his own time at Yale, had been favored by parental latitude not often associated with early New England. It is recorded that his mother, Temperance Holmes, sent him off to Yale "with a Dutch liquor case containing six large bottles filled with various kinds of strong waters, probably brandy, rum, gin, whisky, doubtless enough to craze a whole class of young bacchanalians."

O. W. Holmes received his A.B., Harvard, at the age of twenty, and his production as class poet stopped the graduation ceremonies for eight minutes, so tumultuous was the applause. He entered upon the study of law but was soon to record that "the temple of the law . . . seems very cold and cheerless about the threshold." At about this time he read an editorial in a New York paper lamenting the decision of the Secretary of the Navy to dismantle the famous frigate *Constitution.* Holmes blew up. He dashed off three verses entitled *Old Ironsides*, sent them to the Boston Daily Advertiser, and was famous from one end of the country to the other within a week. He dryly observed that "there is no form of lead-poisoning which more rapidly and thoroughly pervades the blood and bones and marrow than that which reaches the young author through mental contact with type metal."

Old Ironsides

Ay tear her tattered ensign down!
Long has it waved on high,
And many an eye has danced to see
That banner in the sky;
Beneath it rung the battle shout,
And burst the cannon's roar:—
The meteor of the ocean air
Shall sweep the clouds no more.

Her deck once red with heroes' blood,
Where knelt the vanquished foe,
When winds were hurrying o'er the flood
And waves were white below,
No more shall feel the victor's tread,
Or know the conquered knee:—
The harpies of the shore shall pluck
The eagle of the sea!

Oh, better that her shattered hulk
Should sink beneath the wave;
Her thunders shook the mighty deep,
And there should be her grave:
Nail to the mast her holy flag,
Set every threadbare sail,
And give her to the god of storms,
The lightning and the gale!

—Oliver Wendell Holmes

Holmes began to attend lectures at the Massachusetts General Hospital, and heard there the famous "phrenologist" and neuro-anatomist Spurzheim—himself a student investigator of an earlier era. Spurzheim died in the hospital of a "fever" and Holmes was among those who attended the autopsy. He was obviously missing nothing in his new calling.

Holmes the versifier kept up his doggerel for a time, as the poem on Page 150 suggests.

The leaders of the profession in Boston were in the habit of sending their sons abroad for a year's study while undergraduates—a liberal New England tradition which needs reviving on a national scale. John Collins Warren, the surgeon whose name was later to be linked with ether anaesthesia, Nathaniel Bowditch, the navigator and scholar, and James Jackson, the physician-teacher, all sent their sons to Paris. So it was that in March of 1833 Holmes sailed to join them, and set himself up in the pension in which Charlotte Corday had murdered the Revolutionary figure Marat in his bath.

But the flamboyant Holmes of the Hasty Pudding Society was beginning to change. He joined the great teacher Pierre Charles Alexandre Louis on the wards of La Pitié every morning from 7:30 to 10 o'clock. He and James Jackson, Jr., were given the rare privilege of free access to Louis' wards and they, along with Henry Bowditch, passed the stiff examinations necessary to enter "La Societé Médicale d'Observation," over which Louis presided. The weekly meetings were compulsory and brought together young men such as Marshall Hall from England, Chomel, and Gabriel Andral, the 33-year old heir apparent to the chair of medicine. Holmes began to construct in his mind two theories: that most medicines given patients were better given to the fish in the sea; and that puerperal fever could be infectious.

Financially, Holmes put up a running fight with his father and delayed his return to Boston until Christmas, 1835. By then he had visited most of Europe's great medical museums, including that of the physician Boerhaave, in Leyden, no doubt to please old Dr. Waterhouse who had graduated there. But it was the spirit of the great Louis which transfixed him. Louis' charm stemmed from his "modesty in the presence of nature." Louis'

"I am too much in earnest for either humility or vanity, but I do entreat those who hold the keys of life and death to listen to me also for this once. I ask no personal favor, but I beg to be heard in behalf of the women whose lives are at stake, until some stronger voice shall plead for them."

"I trust that I have made the issue perfectly distinct and intelligible. And let it be remembered that this is no subject to be smoothed over by nicely adjusted phrases of half assent and half censure divided between the parties. . . . persons are nothing in this matter; better that twenty pamphleteers should be silenced or as many professors unseated, than that one mother's life should be taken. There is no quarrel here between men, but there is deadly incompatibility and exterminating warfare between doctrines. . . . Indifference will not do here; our journalists and committees have no right to take up their pages with minute anatomy and tediously detailed cases while it is a question whether or not the "black death" of child-bed is to be scattered broadcast by the agency of the mother's friend and advisor. Let the men who mould opinions look to it; if there is any voluntary blindness, any interested oversight, any culpable negligence, even, in such a matter, and the facts shall reach the public ear, the pestilence-carrier of the lying-in chamber must look to God for pardon, for man will never forgive him."

—O. W. Holmes
"The Contagiousness of Puerperal Fever"

"Society for Medical Observation" had claimed Holmes' loyalty. The object of the Society, as he expressed it, was "to make the problems clear to those who took part in it, to teach them to conquer the difficulties, to make observation really useful by making it exact and precise, and finally to show how one can safely proceed from particular facts to sound generalizations." As we shall see, these were the very methods which Holmes soon applied to the scandal of childbed fever in America. To repeat Pasteur's dictum, "fortune favors the prepared mind"—and the world owes much to the mind prepared so well by Pasteur's compatriot P. C. A. Louis.

Before leaving Paris Holmes wrote to his family of what we may regard as some of his "discoveries"—"I have more fully learned at least three principles since I have been in Paris: not to take authority when I can have facts; not to guess when I can know; not to think a man must take physic because he is sick." "My aim has been to qualify myself . . . not for a mere scholar, for a follower after other men's opinions, for a dependent on their authority—but for the character of a man who has seen and therefore knows; who has thought and therefore has arrived at his own conclusions."

On returning to Boston Holmes wrote his M.D. thesis on his observations on "Acute Pericarditis" and graduated M.D. Harvard on February 11, 1836. The influence of Louis carried Holmes forward for another two years of writing as he took the Boylston Essay Prizes for 1836 and 1837 on Malaria in New England, and on Physical Methods in the Medical Examination.

Soon after graduation Holmes joined The Boston Society for Medical Improvement, doubtless to fill the void in his intellectual life previously filled by the little Society in Paris. At one of the Boston meetings he heard of the death of a physician who had assisted at an autopsy a week previously on a woman dead of childbed fever. During the intervening week—the last week of his life—the physician had attended several women in childbirth, and all of these had come down with puerperal sepsis and fever.

This information, coming upon his earlier undergraduate musings in Paris on this subject, produced another outburst of the "Old Ironsides" type. The echo reached to Philadelphia where

"So of your questions, don't in mercy try
To pump your patient absolutely dry;
He's not a mollusk squirming in a dish,
You're not Agassiz, and he's not a fish.

"If the poor victim needs must be percussed,
Don't make an anvil of his aching bust;
(Doctors exist within a hundred miles
Who thump a thorax as they'd hammer piles;)
If you must listen to his doubtful chest,
Catch the essentials and ignore the rest."

—O. W. Holmes
Dean, Harvard Medical School
1847-1853.

the pride of the profession retorted with the haughtiness which characterizes occasionally some figures who are afflicted with "decerebrate rigidity." Thereupon Holmes became the prosecuting attorney in the case, and the sharpening of his wits achieved through his early legal training came to the fore.

In 1842 Holmes became widely known for his paper on "Homeopathy and its kindred delusions." Then, in 1843, with a large part of the profession aware of his keen ability and of his ruthless castigation of sham and fraud in the field of disease, Holmes fired the blast of his career straight at the opposition. In 27 blistering pages of the little-known *New England Quarterly Journal of Medicine and Surgery* he held the mirror up to the obstetricians of the country. Using the methods learned in Paris under Louis he assembled the most damaging case-histories which have ever been printed—not a few, but dozens of them—frightful, nauseating and accurate.

The boy who had stopped Harvard's Convocation ceremonies with his wit and daring had now become the man—able to stop the obstetricians dispensing the foulest disease in the book. Pitifully, physicians wrote to him telling of cases they had lost and now knew why. The personal threats to Holmes only served to intensify the truth of his statements—which could stand on their own merits anywhere. One law-student-turned-physician had cleaned up childbed fever in America. What was his counterpart doing in Europe?

Ignaz Semmelweis was entering the University of Pesth to study philosophy, literature and classics as Holmes was returning to Boston from his Paris sojourn. Born into a shopkeeper's family, the fourth of eight children, Semmelweis determined that he would someday get a university education—if only to counteract the poor schooling he had at home in a rural district forgotten by the Austrian rulers. After two years of what he considered poor lectures at the University of Pesth, he started out at the age of 19 for the University of Vienna where he enrolled in law. After a year in this faculty, however, he determined on medicine and took his first year of it in Vienna. He came to know the great clinician Skoda and the pathologist Rokitansky, men who were later to defend him.

The second and third years of medicine he took at the University of Pesth, returning to Vienna to complete his final year. As an undergraduate there he did research on the supposed value of tartar emetic on pneumonia, working out part of the problem, in rabbits, with Jankowich. The results were not world-shaking in the field of pneumonia, but his apprenticeship in the field of transmitted infection was to bear fruit later.

While Holmes was reaping the whirlwind from his publication on childbed fever of 1843, Semmelweis was completing his medical course, and writing his thesis on "De Vita Plantarum." Because of special courses taken in obstetrics he was able to graduate as both Doctor of Medicine, in April, 1844, and as Doctor of Midwifery in August of the same year.

Semmelweis was aged 28 when he was taken on the First Obstetrical Service of the Allgemeines Krankenhaus as an Assistant. He was shocked to see students coming directly from the dissecting rooms of anatomy and post-morten rooms of pathology into the obstetrical wards where they made vaginal examinations on expectant mothers. He observed that, in contrast, the Second Obstetrical Service, staffed entirely by midwives rather than doctors had a much lower maternal mortality. From his own ward he followed many cases to autopsy, and developed the thesis that they succumbed in all cases to "blood poisoning." When his close friend Kolletschka died of a generalized infection which spread from a dissection wound suffered at an autopsy, Semmelweis felt sure that his surmise was correct that students and physicians were transporting infection from the autopsy room to the women confined on his ward, with fatal results.

Semmelweis started the careful scrubbing of hands with calcium chloride and the cleaning of the delivery room meticulously with this substance. He started to learn English in order to read the papers of Charles White, Gordon, and other British pioneers in this field. Before he began his new antiseptic regime the mortality on his ward was 9.92 per cent, and that on the midwives' ward was 1.33 per cent. Within a year he brought the mortality rate in his ward down to 3.8 per cent. He was merely an Assistant, and could not control the practitioners using the ward. Soon he had the maternal mortality rate down to 1.27 per cent, and passed one summer month, when infection was normally high, without a single death.

At the age of 29, therefore, he told a meeting of the Vienna Medical Society that he believed transmitted infection and resultant blood poisoning was the basis of fatal "puerperal fever." This was too much for "the great" in obstetrics in Vienna and they started an underhanded and vicious persecution of this supposed "upstart." Hebra and Skoda jumped to his defence, aged though they were. In March, 1849, his Assistantship expired and he was barred from the wards and even from his own case records. Scanzoni and the orthodox of that day froze him out, as their counterparts forty years later in the same medical society were to freeze out Freud. Semmelweis was not up against evidence but authority.

The Vienna General Hospital in 1850 further sought to ridicule this life-saving innovator by appointing him "Privat-Dozent for theoretic midwifery with restriction to the use of the phantom and cadaver in his teaching." With this final insult Semmelweis left Vienna forever, and moved to a city hospital in Budapest. Here, because the chief obstetrician was also the chief surgeon there was no shortage of childbed fever. In his first year there Semmelweis reduced the mortality rate to 0.85 per cent. At the end of six years he was able to show that there had been only 8 deaths in 933 patients.

At the age of 37 he succeeded Professor Birly in the Chair of Obstetrics in the University of Pesth, and found the obstetrical ward to be situated between the morgue and the cemetery—both geographically and figuratively. By introducing his antiseptic methods Semmelweis reduced the mortality to 2 deaths in 514 cases. Within two years he started to write the book which made him immortal: *Die Aetiologie der Begrift und die Prophylaxis des Kindbettfiebers.* Published in 1860 the book's introduction sounds a new clear note in European obstetrics:

> My Doctrine is not firmly established in order that the book expounding it may moulder in the dust of a library; my Doctrine has a mission and that is to bring blessings into practical social life.

My Doctrine is produced in order that it may be disseminated by teachers of midwifery, until all who practice medicine, down to the last village doctor and the last village midwife may act according to its principles; my Doctrine is produced in order to banish error from the lying-in hospitals, to preserve the wife to the husband, the mother to the child.

At the age of 47 Semmelweis died in an insane asylum, beaten in body but not in spirit by "the right people" in the wrong century. Today this Hungarian peasant is memorialized by a statue in Elizabeth Square in Budapest, and by a monument in the gardens of the General Hospital in Vienna.

Thus, one hundred years ago, did a Boston poet and a Budapest peasant, both truants from the study of law, change the world for all future mothers.

INFLAMMATION

John Hunter (1728-1793)
Rudolf Virchow (1821-1902)

It is scarcely credible that the immortal John Hunter could neither read nor write at the age of seventeen, that he should be a furniture maker at the age of twenty, and yet, by age forty, be the teacher of Jenner of vaccination fame, and the surgeons Abernethy, Cline, and Astley Cooper, than whom there have been none greater.

Why was this so? Why was John Hunter as averse to schooling in his boyhood as Semmelweis was to be? Writing in his maturity Hunter said: "When I was a boy I wanted to know about the clouds and the grasses, and why the leaves changed colour in the autumn; I watched the ants, bees, birds, tadpoles and cadis worms; I pestered people with questions about what nobody knew or cared anything about."

Hunter spent his life doing just this, albeit in more formal settings; but nevertheless he sought explanations for things long glossed over in ignorance or buried in a fog of theory. As a teacher he built up a corps of patient but implacable enquirers, such as Jenner. In this manner he influenced medicine and surgery for a century after his death in 1793.

One year before he died John Hunter completed his great work of 715 pages, "A treatise on the blood, inflammation and gun-shot wounds." After the dedication of the volume to the King, Hunter wrote: "The following pages, treating of inflammation, were first arranged in the year 1762, at Belle Isle, after the complete reduction of that place. They were compiled from notes and memorandums of observations, made in the course of twelve years' residence in London. During this space my time was occupied partly in my education under the late Dr. William Hunter, and partly in assisting him. In the winter season I was principally employed in the dissecting-room, where I taught the practical part of anatomy; in the summers I attended the hospitals."

Around these facts we can briefly reconstruct John Hunter's early life. He came to London when the furniture-making establishment in Glasgow to which he had been apprenticed was closed. Thus at age twenty he joined his distinguished brother Dr. William Hunter at his Anatomy School in Great Windmill Street. John's adeptness at dissection was a revelation to William, his elder by ten years. Within a year John was preparing all the anatomical demonstrations for William's lectures, and in 1755 he was taken into partnership in the school.

The summers were spent at the Chelsea Hospital attending the practice of the distinguished Cheselden, and later, at St. Bartholomew's Hospital, the practice of Percival Pott. A family scheme to get John to Oxford to study Latin and Greek failed; in his own words—"they wanted to make an old woman of me." He was often to rue his decision, however, for lecturing was to become his greatest opportunity, and yet his greatest trial. (He would take laudanum to settle his stomach before facing his classes.)

However, it was not his early inability to lecture with ease which made him one of the immortals of medicine—who, single-handed, raised surgery up to the status of a great science as well as a distinguished calling. It was the supposed "dreamer" of hilltops rather than desk tops, in rural Scotland, who was now wrestling with the whole of medicine's ignorance, not merely with Hunter's own. It was while he was a student in London that "he began to collect the material for his great work" on inflammation. During his time at St. George's Hospital as a surgeon-pupil Hunter began experiments, later to be recorded in his "Treatise on the blood, inflammation and gun-shot wounds."

Working with furious determination and application he went down with pneumonia. His brother James had succumbed to tuberculosis; John took the warning to heart and cast about for an opportunity to get away on what for him would be a "holiday." This the Army provided for him, sending him to Belle Isle (the small island, midway between Laennec's birthplace, Quimper, and later home, Nantes, in Brittany), which Admiral Hawke took following his destruction of the French fleet in 1759. He later went on with the Army to the Peninsula and remained there until 1763, when he returned to London to enter practice. No Army ever contributed more to scientific surgery through the retention of an experimenter. Hunter's writings on gunshot wounds, inflammations, pyemia, and shock have become classics. Little did the British Army realize that one of its surgeons would also contribute studies on digestion during hibernation in lizards and snakes, and on hearing in fishes!

Our discussion of Hunter ends with his return from the Army, with his student observations finally written up for the first time in a busy life, with invaluable experience of war wounds chronicled, and with the "salutary" influence of inflammation clearly in mind. He wrote: "Inflammation is not only occasionally the cause of diseases, but it is often a mode of cure, since it frequently produces a resolution of indurated parts, by changing the diseased action into a salutary one, if capable of resolution. By these extensive powers *inflammation becomes the first principle in surgery*." (Authors' italics.)

Thus we leave young John Hunter at the age of thirty-five, proud, competent, ever enquiring, forging the new sciences of experimental pathology and surgical pathology with his own two hands. His subsequent rise to the greatest heights ever attained in renown, respect and recognition in the field of medicine needs no retelling here. He made his own opportunities and made medicine great.

Rudolf Virchow (1821-1902)

Fifty years after John Hunter's death, a Pomeranian youth,

Rudolph Virchow, graduated in medicine in Berlin. His life was to change our whole way of thinking about disease; he was to overthrow the speculative theories of humors, vapors and spontaneous generation, and to show that each and every cell derives from an antecedent cell (omnis cellula e cellula).

Who was this layer of new medical foundations, this arch-enemy of Bismarck, this digger-up of Troy?

Virchow began his medical studies at the training establishment for Army surgeons in the Kaiser Wilhelm Akademie, at the age of eighteen. Four years later he graduated with the medical degree of the University of Berlin. His student thinking was greatly influenced by that great spirit, Johannes Müller, of whom he later wrote: "There is no school of Müller in the sense of dogmas, for he taught none, but only in the sense of methods."

In this liberal atmosphere Virchow was to start thinking for himself. Strangely his thoughts turned to inflammation, and in Hunterian fashion he went to the heart of the matter, oblivious of the doctrines which had inhibited thought in this field since Hunter's great work.

As a second year medical student we find Virchow writing home to his father, asking him to set aside some rabbits for his experimental work. His Latin thesis, presented in 1843, for his graduation in medicine, was entitled, "De rheumate praesertim corneae." His distinguished biographer, Erwin Ackerknecht, has written: "The fact that Virchow did research here on inflammation in a nonvascular tissue determined in a way all his later opinions on parenchymatous inflammation, and therewith on the cellular, and not vascular basis of inflammation."

Upon graduation Virchow was enabled to carry on his work on inflammation thanks to a prosectorship at the Charité Hospital under the distinguished Froriep. At the age of twenty-five Virchow fired his first warning rocket before the Berlin Society for Scientific Medicine in a paper entitled "Points of View in Scientific Medicine." He published this in the first volume of *The Archive for Pathological Anatomy and Physiology and for Clinical Medicine*, which he founded with his friend Reinhardt, and which for brevity has ever since been called *Virchow's Archiv.* The paper might as well have been entitled "Death for dogmatism," so trenchant were the criticisms of the philosophical systems which had strangled experiment in the field of normal and diseased states. He issued a call for help to the other natural sciences. He concluded: "Let us not deceive ourselves about the condition of medicine. Minds are unmistakably exhausted by the many hypothetical systems again and again cast aside only to be replaced by new ones. A few more invasions perhaps and this time of unrest will have passed by and it will be recognized that only quiet, industrious and persevering work, the true work of observation or experiment, possesses enduring value. Pathological physiology will then gradually be developed, not as the production of a few heated brains, but as the work of many patient investigators; that pathological physiology, which is the citadel of scientific medicine, of which pathological anatomy and the clinic are only out-works."

In 1848, an explosive year in Europe, with the *Communist Manifesto* of Marx and Engels abroad in the land, Virchow was sent to Silesia to investigate the causes of a serious typhus epidemic. His report was so scathing a denunciation of social and sanitary conditions there, that the Prussian Government began to wonder if its hour had come. It was not accustomed to being berated in the name of freedom, democracy and justice in its public health reports. Accordingly Virchow was dismissed from his position in Berlin.

In Wurzburg he found a congenial atmosphere for his researches and there pressed his work on inflammation to the full, with his able pupils. He began also to generalize from the botanists' "Cell theory" to the field of pathology. After seven years' exile he was invited back to Berlin by the unanimous vote of the medical faculty and there began his work on "The cellular pathology" as his great volume of 1858 was called. The Prussian Government even built him a Pathological Institute.

Virchow sat in the Reichstag for many years, taught the medical students, conducted a large research programme, fought the anti-vivisectionists, provided Berlin with an adequate sewage system * and hammered away at Bismarck. Sherrington often

* Georges Fernand Widal (1862-1929) born in Algiers, began his work on typhoid fever with Chantemesse in Paris a year prior to graduation. The Widal agglutination test—in the diagnosis of typhoid fever—is in daily use still throughout the world.

recalled his visit to the Reichstag with Virchow, and of seeing Bismarck emerge from a door high up, like a cuckoo from a clock, to chastise the members below.

Anthropology was one of Virchow's great interests and he assisted Schliemann in the discoveries unearthed at Troy. When, after an absence of ten years, Osler returned to Berlin he carried with him four fine examples of Indian skulls from British Columbia for his old teacher, Virchow identified their origin at once.

The world has seen but rarely such all-embracing medical scientists as John Hunter and Rudolf Virchow. Hunter's famous statement to Jenner epitomizes much of his philosophy: "But why think, why not try the experiment. Be patient. Be accurate."

Virchow's motto might well have been, "Ohne hast, ohne rast." He knew the value of application to a broad, basic problem, such as inflammation—which occupied him from his second year of medical school until he became absorbed in cellular pathology fifteen years later. He knew also the value of grit and determination in a new field, and he lived to see his work and himself not merely recognized, but idolized. As we leave him we must quote his prophetic words, written in his thirties: "There are also those who, if they do not create the current, still give to it its direction and force. These men are not always the happiest. Many go down in the movement, or by it. Many grow weary after they have given to it their best forces. Much power and great tenacity are necessary if the individual shall not only live to see his triumph but also to enjoy it."

Sir James Paget (1814-1899)

Every medical student knows that two diseases were named after Paget—*osteitis deformans* with the shortening of the long bones and enlargement of the head, and *Paget's disease of the nipple*, a surface cancer. What first year students do not realize perhaps is that one in their position in 1835 discovered the true nature of the "bony spicules" encountered, in those days, in the muscles of cadavers being dissected.

Paget described his discovery of the pork parasites in humans thus: "Another event in this first year's study, which had some influence on my later life, was the discovery of the *Trichina spiralis*. Dr. Cobbold has told the story of the several steps leading to the discovery and following it, in his latest work on the *Entozoa*. My share was the detection of the 'worm' in its capsule; and I may justly ascribe it to the habit of looking-out, and observing, and wishing to find new things, which I had acquired in my previous studies of botany. All the men in the dissecting-rooms, teachers included, 'saw' the little specks in the muscles: but I believe that I alone 'looked at' them and observed them: no one trained in natural history could have failed to do so."

But this is only part of the story. Paget was one of seventeen children and his father, a provisioner of the Royal Navy at Yarmouth at the Battle of Camperdown, had lost his business by the time James was ready for medical school. As a result, an apprenticeship was entered into with a Yarmouth practitioner, which did not speed James' medical education, but it gave him time to botanize with his brother Charles. Together they published a little volume in 1834, "A sketch of the natural history of Yarmouth and its neighborhood." James was able to draw well and he was conscientious in his identification and labelling of all the specimens which they collected. Thus, in addition to seeing patients, dispensing, running messages and keeping accounts, he learned, above all, method.

By borrowing enough money from a brother student Paget was able to pay his fees at St. Bartholomew's Hospital medical school, entering in October, 1834. Having taught himself French and German he was able to translate for his teacher, Marshall Hall, the latest papers of Johannes Müller on reflex action in the nervous system. He headed his class in his first year in medicine, surgery, chemistry and botany!

His discovery of the true nature of the parasites found in the muscles dissected was no mere accident. He had to work at it, as we shall see. He was determined to examine "the little specks" with a microscope, but there was no microscope in the entire hospital! He therefore, through a letter of introduction, visited the head of the Natural History department of the British Museum, who, it became clear, had no microscope either. Finally, Paget sought out the head of the Botany section there, by whom he was loaned a microscope with which to discover the little worms

—curled up, and by now probably smiling, in their protective capsules.

To condense and complete the story of this great clinician we may say that he became "serjeant surgeon to the Queen," a great pathologist, the chronicler and educator par excellence of St. Bartholomew's Hospital, one of the founders of The Queen's Institute of District Nursing, and Vice-Chancellor of the University of London.

Paget was one of the first medical educators to keep adequate records on the progress of his students after graduation. He was a pungent lecturer, as witness the following reference to some surgeons in his paper, "The Calamities of Surgery": "They make their brains like sieves, and they run all the little things through and retain all the big ones which they suppose to be their successes; and a very mischievous heap of rubbish it is that they retain."

Paget, fortunately for medicine, lived in an era in which all disciplines or callings within this branch of science could still speak to each other in an understandable language. The horizon had not yet been darkened by the gibberish and the tortured verbal emesis of a later day. It was therefore possible for Paget, in his Croonian Lecture before the Royal Society in 1857, "On the causes of the rhythmic motion of the heart," to put before Hughlings Jackson the suggestion that "the time-regulated rhythmic action, whether of the nervous centre or of the independent contractile walls is due to their nutrition being rhythmic." Jackson immediately grasped the significance of this hypothesis for his studies in the nervous system and used it to develop his views on the periodicity of epileptic seizures.

Paget's discovery, his apprenticeship in natural history, his labors in pathology, his clinical acumen and love of teaching, we shall see echoed in the life of William Osler.

William Osler (1849-1919)

Thousands of cars course along the highway hourly between Hamilton and Dundas, Ontario. No one in them sees anything remarkable about the little pools and springs beside the road. Yet it was with a study of the microscopic creatures within one such spring that the ink-pot career of William Osler began. His little paper, "Christmas and the Microscope," appeared in Hardwicke's Science-Gossip, London, 1869, and like so many papers and addresses to follow, it began with a quotation—this one from Horace.

It is hard to believe that a boy scraping the algae off the sides of a barrel with a stick on this December afternoon would some day write the world's greatest textbook of medicine and inspire the two largest medical foundations ever created. His influence on medical education was world-wide, and his contribution to the literature and history of medicine unequalled in modern times.

Osler was raised in a country manse, one of nine children. Though given to wild escapades as a child he became a close student of nature under the Rev. W. A. Johnson, the godson of the Duke of Wellington, at Trinity College School at Weston, Ontario. The physician to the School, Dr. James Bovell, stimulated Osler's interest in nature and was later to shepherd him into Trinity College Medical School at Toronto, where he was Dean. The study of fossils, the grinding of bones and teeth, and the microscopic examination of all manner of water dwellers kept Osler busy. School for him was a mixture of athletics and scientific investigation, though a great knowledge of the classics was to rub off on him.

Entering Trinity College, Toronto, in theology, Osler eventually transferred to the study of medicine and his naturalist's eye soon fell on the minute cysts of the pork parasite, *Trichina spiralis*, in the muscles of the cadaver which he was dissecting. From one drachm of arm muscle he isolated 159 cysts, most of which contained live worms, moving sluggishly. These parasites had been discovered and first described in 1835 by James Paget when a first year medical student in London.

Osler tried to infect animals with these, testing dogs, cats and rabbits, being successful only in the rabbits. He pursued the subject with the help of a veterinary hospital in Toronto, and then put his data aside, to attend to his medical course. (He drew on these undergraduate researches when in 1876 he gave the Somerville Lectures in Montreal.)

In the same year (1870) Osler compiled his observations on

"Canadian Diatomaceae" and published a first class paper on them, listing 109 species in 29 genera, found mostly in the Dundas marshlands.

Migrating to McGill Medical Faculty in 1870 because of the clinical facilities of the Montreal General Hospital, Osler became even further immersed in his undergraduate ink-pot career. In the tradition of the *Lancet*, the *Canadian Medical and Surgical Journal* published, under "Hospital Practice," an account of interesting cases appearing on the hospital wards. The clinical clerks wrote up such reports, Osler, in two years, having six printed. The subjects were: suppurative nephritis, fissure of anus, angina Ludovici, carcinoma mammae, pleuropneumonia with delirium tremens (Osler doing the autopsy and demonstrating a large renal infarct). Dr. John Reddy read a paper before the Montreal Medico-Chirurgical Society on paralysis with aphasia, in which the post mortem specimen was prepared by Osler, neatly showing the offending blood clot in the arteries of the brain. Meanwhile his old Toronto hobby of parasites was carried on.

For his graduation in 1872 Osler prepared such a thesis as is rarely seen. It was a report on fifty post mortems. The Faculty were so impressed with its "originality and research" together with the 33 microscopic and other preparations accompanying it, that they awarded Osler a special prize.

Only the introduction to his thesis survives, but it is written with such sweep and imagination as to be worthy of quotation here:

> In that Trinity of being—of body mind and soul—which so marvellously make up the Man, each one has its own special ills and diseases. With the first of these—the body—have we here anything to do, leaving the second to be attended to by that class of men whose duty it is, "to minister to minds diseased," i.e. the Psychologists, while those of the third class beyond a Physician's skill seek aid elsewhere. Few indeed are permitted to end their days in a natural manner, by a gradual decline of the vital powers, till that point reached, where nutrition failing to supply the fuel, necessary to keep the lamp of life alight, leaves decay to drag back the fabric to the dust. . . . The number of avenues through which death may reach us, the natural frailty of our bodies the delicate

and intricate machinery which maintains us in a condition of health may well make us exclaim with the Poet

> Strange that a harp of thousand strings
> Should keep in tune so long.

To investigate the causes of death, to examine carefully the condition of organs, after such changes have gone on in them as to render existence impossible and to apply such Knowledge to the prevention and treatment of disease, is one of the highest objects of the Physician.

We are not surprised that within a year Osler had made in London an important discovery on the rôle of the "platelets" of the blood.

Osler's eventual rise to the Chair of Medicine in the new Johns Hopkins Hospital Medical School in 1888 and his translation to the Regius Professorship of Medicine at Oxford in 1905 need no retelling, thanks to the labors of Harvey Cushing, whose *Life of Sir William Osler* is one of the classics of our language. Suffice it to say that the world has not known Osler's equal as a teacher, writer, speaker and, above all, physician. His three score years and ten (1849-1919) were some of the most momentous in the history of discovery. Through the felicity of Cushing's pen they have been preserved for generations who succeeded Osler.

David Gruby (1810-1898)

For success in overcoming a veritable jungle of obstacles to a medical career few students compare with David Gruby. This son of a Hungarian farmer with eight children was raised in a village where, as Kisch relates in his admirable memoir, juvenile delinquents were marked for public notice by having their teeth broken off by the farrier with his horseshoeing instruments!

Early in life Gruby was apprenticed to a lens-grinder and watchmaker. At the age of fifteen he set off on foot for Pesth, the capital of Hungary, with twenty-five cents and a loaf of bread from his father. In Pesth, he supported himself as a bookkeeper to a small restaurant. The Piarist Gymnasium was the best school in the city but was closed to Jews, so that David, having selected it for its high standards, sought an education there by the process of sitting outside the classroom door. One of the teachers, on observing such determination, took him into his classes despite the rules.

At the age of twenty-one Gruby had accumulated enough money, as he thought, and sufficient background learning to enter the faculty of medicine in Vienna University. To supplement his savings he tutored other students, living all the while in "Eagle Street" in the Latin Quarter—in the turreted house in which, legend has it, the famous Paracelcus lived three hundred years before and by his genius transmuted pennies into gold with which to pay his landlord! This story of Aureolus Theophrastus Bombastus von Hohenheim is probably as factual as most of his remedies.

Gruby lacked any such alchemy, though he had a little chemical laboratory high in the turret. He lived on potatoes for weeks on end, reminiscent of J. S. Billings' diet as a student in Cincinnati. Gruby's first examinations were so successfully passed that he was exempted from paying further tuition fees.

He was so anxious to investigate various body fluids that he built himself a microscope in 1835. Later his teacher Rokitansky allowed him to use a good one—a Ploessl—which permitted observations by daylight. After years of independent work, and of encouragement by the pathologist Rokitansky and the anatomist Berres, Gruby published his doctoral thesis, "The Morphology of Pathological Fluids," with 103 illustrations by his own hand. This work brought him great acclaim for it was really the first publication in which the microscopic differences in pus cells were ascribed to differences in the diseases themselves. Gruby described the destructive effect of distilled water on white blood cells used to a saline habitat, and the effect of acetic acid in making more clearly visible the nuclei of white cells—a procedure used in every hospital laboratory today. Coagulation of the blood and the formation of new capillaries in inflamed tissue were also discussed. In many ways Gruby's student work was a counterpart of Virchow's undergraduate investigation.

Gruby soon came to official notice of a most favorable kind and he was offered a professorship in Vienna University if he would become a Christian. Sir William Bowman placed him in the same class as Purkinje, the great Czech contributor to medical science. Gruby became interested in nutrition and in the role of electrolytes. Like Virchow he investigated sources of disease and compaigned for the filtering of the Vienna water supply for poor and rich alike.

On the suggestion of Roux, Dupuytren's successor at Hôtel Dieux in Paris, Gruby settled in the French capital and lived there until his death fifty-eight years later. One of his first activities in his new home was to develop a pathological service at the Foundling Hospital, where the structural and chemical abnormalities of the newborn could be studied. A group of foreign physicians studying in Paris suggested that Gruby give them systematic lectures in this field, and in time Gruby came to number among his pupils, Frederic Berg of Stockholm, Milne-Edwards, Claude Bernard, Flourens and even Magendie. In Paris Gruby began his microscopic studies on skin diseases for which he is famous today, and as in the case of modern dermatologists he was a pioneer in new photographic methods. He discovered the cause of favus, a fungus disease of the skin, contagious in nature, the *microsporum*, the fungi *trichophyton tonsurans*, and *oidium albicans*, the cause of thrush.

Daniel Carrion (1859-1885)

Daniel Carrion has a special place among undergraduate contributors to medical science—he paid with his life for his belief in the transmission of the disease known as *Verruga Peruana*.

He was born in Cerro de Pasco, Peru, in 1859, the son of a physician-lawyer from Ecuador. His mother was of Peruvian stock. The boy was always small in stature but popular with his schoolmates and teachers. He had a distinguished record in his secondary schooling at the Collegio National de Guadalupe. He studied the physical and natural sciences at the Universidad Mayo de San Marco. In 1880 he entered the Medical Faculty of San Fernando, now known as the Faculty of Carrion. His clinical training was taken in the Dos de Mayo and San Bartolome hospitals.

The setting for Carrion's student discovery is interesting. An earlier medical student, Salazar, in 1858 presented a graduation thesis on the "Historia de las Verrugas," in which he held that the disease was water-borne, and that a late skin eruption heralded a fatal outcome. The disease, since the time of "the conquest" had been likened in its virulence to "the pest." More recently, during the year of 1870 to be exact, the disease had taken the lives of 7,000 workers who were building the Trans-Andean Railroad in the final section from Callao to the terminal in Oroya. With such losses, it was natural that there should be much speculation as to the spread of the disease. The natives could not understand how a disease which produced nothing visible except "warts" could be fatal. In fact, many thought that Oroya fever had nothing to do with Peruvian warts.

When a fourth-year student, Carrion addressed himself to this interesting and obviously practical problem. He spent his vacation in assembling case histories of victims of the disease, and made a map showing their geographical distribution. He found that only near Oroya was the disease endemic.

On the clinical side he found that running through all the cases there was a sequence of events. Strong Chilean workers, used to an altitude of 6,500 feet, were usually taken with a severe fever, a profound weakness, joint pains, anaemia and leucocytosis. Physicians spoke of it variously as "acute pernicious anaemia," and as atypical malaria. Some blamed it on the hot springs. No one could explain its existence in the Huarochiri region of the Oroya route. For some reason there was general agreement that verruga could not be transmitted by inoculation.

On August 27, 1885, against the entreaties of his associates, Daniel Carrion had a friend inoculate him with blood from a 14-year old boy who had been admitted to hospital with the typical Verruga Peruana skin eruption. Carrion was going to prove or disprove the connection between Oroya fever and Verruga Peruana. For three weeks he was buoyant and well, but on September 19th he began to have intermittent muscular pains followed by prostration. His red blood corpuscles fell to 1,085,000 per cubic millimetre, and became distorted. On October 5, 1885, he died—38 days after the inoculation. The post mortem which was done shed a great deal of light on the manner of spread of the disease throughout the body and on the end results of the infection. Carrion's question of the connection between the two "diseases" was answered.

Thus, at the age of 26, another medical student contributor was listed among the missing. Many hospitals and dispensaries in Latin America have been named in Carrion's honour and not least of all, his old faculty itself.

William George MacCallum (1874-1944)

W. G. MacCallum, the older brother of J. B. MacCallum (p. 63), was born in Dunnville, Ontario, April 18, 1874. His father was a general practitioner with a great love of natural history. The brothers MacCallum spent a considerable amount of time in the improvised laboratory which their father had set up behind their home.

At the age of 15, William entered the University of Toronto, determined to specialize in classics. He took up the study of Greek at once, and only on his father's urging did he enroll in courses in Zoology, Chemistry and Physics. In the summers he spent his time botanizing and collecting and he often joined his father in visiting patients in the country.

In 1894, he graduated from the University of Toronto with honours and was still bent on making his mark in the classics. However, his father persuaded him that the recently opened medical school at Johns Hopkins University in Baltimore should be his goal. With considerable misgiving Johns Hopkins admitted him to the medical school with second year status, and this, above all, into their first enrolled class. The misgivings were short lived, however, for on graduation in 1897 W. G. MacCallum led the entire class.

Under the influence of such men as William Osler, William Halsted, and William Welch, MacCallum's bent for developing new and unusual lines of thought flourished. There was abroad in the land a potent new ferment in the form of the Johns Hopkins medical school and MacCallum was the first of a truly remarkable group of men to catch the fire from the brilliant teachers assembled there. As an undergraduate, he made a discovery of very great medical importance. He described for the first time the sexual cycle of the malarial parasite in the crow. His description and interpretation of the phenomenon of flagellation of the malarial parasite was a fundamental step in both tropical and general medicine. It reflected his early training as an observant naturalist. It is of interest that his brother J. B. MacCallum, while convalescing from tuberculosis in Jamaica in 1902, started some work on the relation of the mosquito to malaria. Sir Ronald Ross, who had misinterpreted the flagellated form, wrote later: "I have ever since felt disgraced as a man of science."

On graduation W. G. MacCallum interned for one year at the Johns Hopkins Hospital in Baltimore. He then served his apprenticeship in Pathology under William Welch, becoming Resident in 1901. With his colleague Voegtlin, he succeeded, after five years of ceaseless attention to the problem of tetany, in demonstrating the effect on calcium metabolism of the minute endocrine glands—the parathyroids—described by another student discoverer, Ivar Sandstrom, in Stockholm in 1877 (p. 124).

MacCallum's name would have gone down to posterity on either of his two remarkable discoveries. But in addition to this he became famous for development of "the case method" of teaching pathology. The evolution of his broad and dynamic outlook in the teaching of pathology may have begun in 1908, when he was given a special chair of Pathological Physiology at Columbia University and as Pathologist at the Presbyterian Hospital at New York. When he succeeded to the chair of Pathology at Johns Hopkins in 1917, then vacated by his great teacher William Welch, he set out to develop thinkers in the field of pathology. His *Text Book of Pathology* was unorthodox and successful and influenced teaching methods the world over. Although endowed with an encyclopaedic memory and with the ability to make detail fascinating, he nevertheless had the gift of bringing students along with him, never making them feel small or ignorant before their fellows. He was greatly addicted to the biographical method of teaching and was an early member of the Johns Hopkins Historical Club. There he presented two papers on "Marcello Malpighi" and "The School of Montpellier." Without family attachments, he travelled very widely and was able to enliven his lectures with details about the important centres of learning which he had visited.

He was early known to the students as a collector of photographs of contributors to medicine which he placed in the laboratory corridors. These he brought to life with some engaging descriptive notes such as:

> Robert Fludd (de Fluctibus) 1570-1630?
> Physician in London, contemporary of Bacon and Harvey. Thought warmth and cold the chief forces and related the most important diseases with the direction of the wind. Cause of the disease was sin, its cure prayer. But he invented a thermometer to determine the temperature of the blood.

> A. P. Gasser 1505-1577 Lindau
> Studied in Vienna and at Montpellier. Lived and practised medicine in Avignon and Feldkirchen. Wrote "Curationes et Observationes medica." This is not the discoverer of the Gasserian Ganglion, who was Johann Ludvig Gasser, Professor of Anatomy in Vienna, but neither was he, for it was described by his grateful student, R. B. Hirsch, in an inaugural dissertation, in 1765.

It was little wonder then that when this remarkable teacher of pathology posted the list, in the laboratory, of subjects the history of which might be written, there should be an immediate and enthusiastic response by the students. The industry with which they entered into their side of the arrangement was a reward which MacCallum well merited.

Both with undergraduates and graduate students in his laboratory, MacCallum adopted the theory that they must learn for themselves and either sink or swim. He lived a charmed life with an abiding interest in students, music, and travel, and in an atmosphere innocent of the administrative heartaches of today.

PLATE 6

(a) R. T. H. Laennec (1781-1826). Self portrait. Courtesy the Bettmann Archive, New York.

(b) Title page of Laennec's student paper on peritonitis.

(c) Rudolf Virchow (1821-1902) as a young professor. From: Long, Esmond: *Selected Readings in Pathology*, 1929. Courtesy of Charles C Thomas, Publisher.

(d) William Stokes at the age of forty-five. From: Major, Ralph: *Classic Descriptions of Disease*, 1932. Courtesy of Charles C Thomas, Publisher.

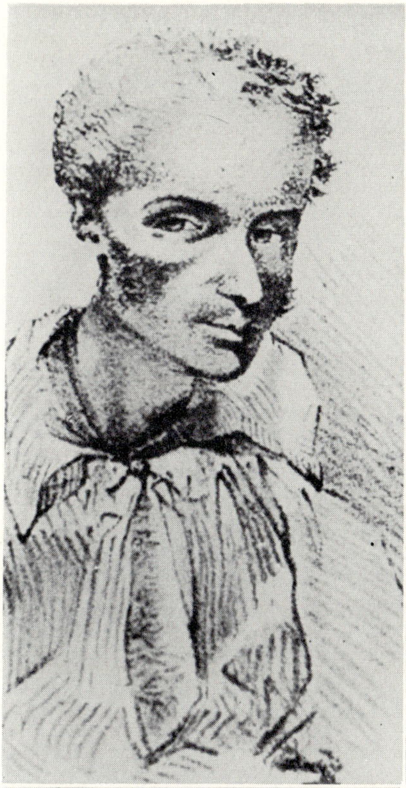

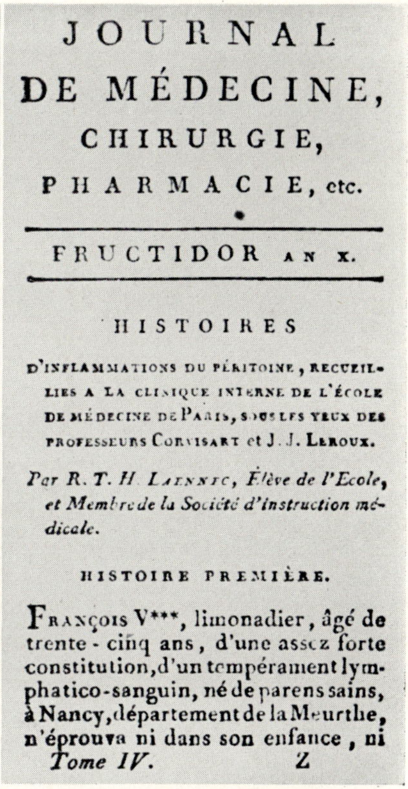

JOURNAL
DE MÉDECINE,
CHIRURGIE,
PHARMACIE, etc.

FRUCTIDOR AN X.

HISTOIRES

D'INFLAMMATIONS DU PÉRITOINE, RECUEILLIES A LA CLINIQUE INTERNE DE L'ÉCOLE DE MÉDECINE DE PARIS, SOUS LES YEUX DES PROFESSEURS CORVISART et J. J. LEROUX.

Par R. T. H. LAENNEC, Élève de l'École, et Membre de la Société d'instruction médicale.

HISTOIRE PREMIÈRE.

FRANÇOIS V***, limonadier, âgé de trente-cinq ans, d'une assez forte constitution, d'un tempérament lymphatico-sanguin, né de parens sains, à Nancy, département de la Meurthe, n'éprouva ni dans son enfance, ni

Tome IV. Z

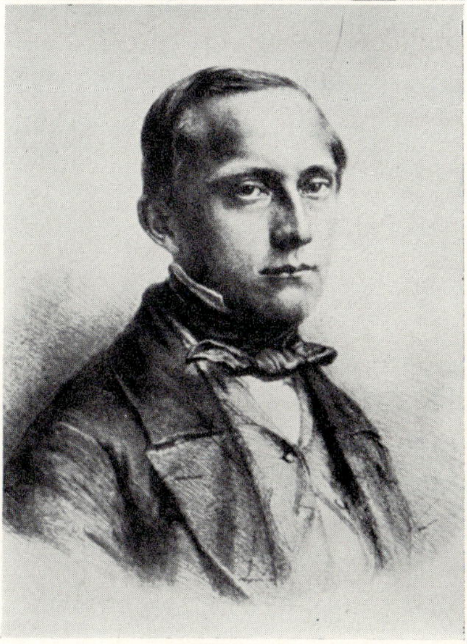

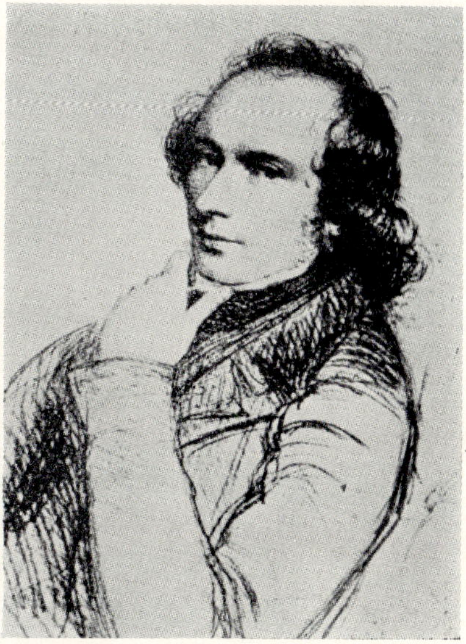

←

Chapter IX

The Lymphatics

BASIC DISCOVERIES in the anatomy of the lymph circulation of the body were made by three medical students, Pecquet, Rudbeck and Joyliffe, independently, and almost simultaneously. This fact has been obscured regrettably by squabbles over priority between one of the students, Rudbeck the Swede, and Professor Thomas Bartholin of Copenhagen. For our purposes the priority issue is of little importance. One could scarcely wish for a better demonstration of student originality and independence of thought than that demonstrated by the following young pioneers.

Jean Pecquet (1622-1674)

Jean Pecquet of Dieppe and Paris, studied medicine at Montpellier. He came under the influence of Vesling, the anatomist, who, like Aselli of Cremona, had already seen the lacteals, or lymph-bearing vessels, of the intestine. In 1647 or 1648 Pecquet left what he called "that mute and frigid science"—anatomy—and in the Vesalian temper set about the study of living animals. On removing the heart of a dog he noticed some whitish fluid in the pericardium and thought it must be pus. On further investigation, however, he found that it issued from the superior vena cava and that abdominal pressure increased its flow. Thus he was led to two momentous discoveries. His first was that contrary to the teachings of Aselli the lacteals, in ascending from the intestine, did not enter the liver at all. The second was that the flow was to the receptaculum chyli and through the thoracic duct into the venous system at the junction of the left jugular and the subclavian veins. His systematic method of working out his problem was in the tradition of William Harvey—whose discovery of the circulation of the blood in 1628 had set the stage for just such studies as Pecquet was now making.

Pecquet's findings were independently confirmed by the Dutch anatomist Van Horne in his *Nova ductus chyliferus* (1652). Pecquet's discoveries were published in his *Experimenta Nova anatomica* (Paris, 1651). William Harvey, in a letter to Morison in Paris, in 1652, credits Pecquet with the first demonstration of the thoracic duct and receptaculum chyli.

Harvey's views on the centrifugal nature of the arterial blood flow found a supporter in Pecquet who wrote, of a later set of experiments:

> "I tied the crural artery of the dog, avoiding the vein, and amputating the member a little beyond the ligature. Only a few drops of blood escaped from the divided veins, but there was no haemorrhage.

Pecquet's discoveries were the beginning of the end of Galen's view that the blood was formed in the liver. The fact that the lacteals were now shown to circumvent the liver was something which could be reconciled with Harvey's views on the circulation of the blood. Thomas Bartholin finally accepted Pecquet's views concerning the by-passing of the liver, in his *Vasa lymphatica in humane nuper inventa* (1654).

Olof Rudbeck (1630-1702)

While Pecquet was completing his works for the press, the Swedish medical student Olof Rudbeck in Uppsala was watching the butchering of a calf. He saw a "whey-like fluid" exuding from the supra-clavicular notch, and being an inquisitive student, of twenty years of age, he sought its source. He found what is now known as the thoracic duct, and traced it back to a swollen segment full of a milk-like fluid. His formal medical studies prevented him from further investigating this field until a year later when, in a cat, he was able to demonstrate the flow from the lacteals to the "vesicula chyli" as he called the pooling point, and thence through the thoracic duct into the venous system.

By April of 1652, Rudbeck had made observations on various phases of this problem in four hundred animals, including cats, dogs, sheep, calves, goats and wolves. The movement of fluid away from the liver, rather than to it, was soon established by his use of ligatures. Rudbeck pressed on to investigate the lymph vessels of the rectum, following them to the cysterna chyli; he later traced lymphatics to an oesophageal gland, to the abdominal wall, to glands between the lung and heart, and to the dorsal side of the sternum.

In April, 1652, Rudbeck gave a demonstration of the lymphatics of the liver to Queen Christina of Sweden, before the court and a large assembly of Swedish and foreign university professors. So interested did the Queen become in Rudbeck's work that she later sent him abroad to study. At the Royal demonstration Rudbeck learned for the first time of Pecquet's work, and in June, 1652, one of the Court physicians showed him a copy of Pecquet's publication of 1651. Rudbeck then realized how completely he had confirmed Pecquet's work, even to the discarding of the liver as a blood-forming organ.

In May, 1652, Rudbeck defended his graduation thesis at Uppsala, "De circulatione sanguinis," — in which the Harveian interpretation of the blood's circulation was introduced to Sweden.

In the summer of 1653 Rudbeck's extended observations on the lymphatics were published in his home town of Vesteras, near Uppsala, as *Nova excercitatio anatomica, exhibens ductus hepaticos aquosos et vasa glandularum serosa.*

In rejecting the liver as a blood-forming organ of the body, Rudbeck substituted a cleansing or purifying rôle for it. He wrote:

> Even as ordinary cooking requires not only fire but also kettles, skillets, etc., through which that which is being cooked is purified and freed from scum, so in nature the heart is not alone to be considered. It requires help of other organs; e.g. the spleen for fer-

mentation, the kidneys for freeing from watery parts, and the liver for freeing from bile and the new fluid (lymph). Only after this is complete is the blood serviceable for the nourishment of the body.

While passing through Hamburg on his way to Holland, on August 16, 1653, Rudbeck first saw Thomas Bartholin's work on the lymphatics, published in May of that year. When he reached Leyden, on his post-graduate journey under Queen Christina's patronage, he arranged to have his little book republished by the physician-publisher Hemsterhugs. This publisher was also bringing out a new edition of Thomas Bartholin's Copenhagen paper, *De Lacteis thoracicis in homine brutisque nuperrime observatis*, and for some reason produced the two works, bound together, under the title, *The Golden Harvest of the Last Three Years!* The volume contained the seeds of a future controversy in the form of a letter by Rudbeck suggesting that Bartholin had pre-dated his work falsely. Polemical arguments such as developed were relished by supporters on both sides, and brought the much neglected lymphatic circulation into immediate prominence.

Larsell feels that Hammarsten's summary of the controversy is apt:

> The chief honor due Rudbeck is that he, a young student, completed a work which by wealth of observation, better prepared drawings, a deeper insight into and nearer approach of results, together with great independence in interpretation, and clearer grasp of the meaning of his observations, is thus entitled to greater scientific credit than the same work which under similar circumstances would be done by the learned professor, one of the foremost anatomists of the time.

In Holland Rudbeck succumbed to the attractions of botany, returning after a year's absence to teach botany and medicine at Uppsala. Thus the wheel had come a full circle—for botany, as well an anatomy and physiology, had been taught by Rudbeck's father in Sweden. The father had originally been a Bishop and a professor of theology.

In retrospect Olof Rudbeck's childhood is interesting. He was born tenth in a family of eleven children. At the age of ten he made a clock out of handcarved wooden parts. A year later he made an abortive attempt to enter the University of Uppsala! However, when he did finally enter he became a real observer, and according to Larsell questioned and tested everything—a trait happily found still in some students despite the lock-step educational systems through which many of them pass.

It is not surprising to us that Rudbeck was made Chancellor of the University of Uppsala at the age of thirty-one. Fortunately for science he did not give up his active investigative career, but ventured into astronomy, architecture, the construction of marine compasses and the furtherance of technical education. He built a botanical garden second only to that of Paris, and founded many new laboratories at Uppsala. When hard times came upon the University he was blamed, as presidents are today, for enlarging the university at the expense of the professors' salaries.

His activity was prodigious in the field of botany alone. In 1666 the entire harbarium of Copenhagen, which had been captured by the Swedes, was taken to Uppsala, and there was catalogued by Rudbeck in twelve volumes containing seven thousand plates. Linnaeus named the genus "Rudbeckia" in his honour.

Rudbeck was the scourge of the old scholasticism and poked fun at its devotees in the following manner:

> However primitive was the natural philosophy of the time, yet there were few who would depart from it. . . . With a word it resolved many difficulties without blackening the hands with charcoal in chemistry, neither did one get backache from inquiring into the nature of earths, metals and minerals, nor did the stomach become weak from dissecting, nor the eyes from staying awake nights to observe the peculiarities of the stars, etc., but in a warm house by fictitious words and distinctions, men became learned and he was held most learned who could think in the most subtle manner.

George Joyliffe (1621-1658)

The third member of this triumvirate of student discoverers was George Joyliffe, called by Evelyn in his famous diary (January 10, 1657) "first detector of the lymphatic veins."

Joyliffe was born in 1621 of an old Oxford family then residing in East Stower, Dorset. At the age of sixteen George followed his brother Richard to Wadham College, Oxford. During his three years up at Oxford Joyliffe moved across to Pembroke College, doubtless under the influence of Pembroke's master, Thomas Clayton, who was also Regius Professor of Medicine. It is recorded in the diary of Thomas ã Wood that Joyliffe gave up the Civil War to return to his studies and "entered on the physic line, and exercising himself in anatomy, with the help of Dr. Clayton, Master of his College and the King's Professor of Physic, he made some discovery of that fourth sort of Vessels, plainly differing from veins, arteries and nerves, now called Lymphe-ducts."

Joyliffe, already a B.A. and M.A. of Oxford, in 1650 entered Clare Hall, Cambridge, as a Fellow Commoner studying for the M.D. degree. This he received in 1652, having studied under the great Francis Glisson, then Regius Professor of Physic at Cambridge. In his famous book *Anatomia hepatis* (Amsterdam, 1659) Glisson recalls the history of Joyliffe's earlier observations on the lymphatics:

> I first came upon a notice of them at the instance of Dr. Joyliffe, and that in the year 1652, at the beginning of June; at what time this man who was graduating as a doctor had come to me at Cambridge for that end. He asserted that a fourth kind of vessel was provided, clearly distinct from veins, arteries, and nerves; and that these were distributed to all or at any rate most parts of the body and contained aqueous humours within them. He added further that he had investigated the duct of these same vessels in several animals; in the joints, testicles, uterus and even in other parts; and that he was certainly convinced that the fluid in them made its way inwards towards the mesentery, and especially to its origin or root. I thought it better then to leave the whole of this matter to the first Discoverer for further elucidation.

Joyliffe went to London in 1653 where, according to Wood, "he made a full and open discovery of the said Vasa lymphatica in Anatomy lectures at the College of Physicians." He practised in Garlick Hythe where he numbered Pepys among his patients. He died in 1658.

Charles Darwin (1758-1778)

The first Charles Darwin, uncle of Charles Robert Darwin (1809-1882) the author of *The Origin of Species*, was a later student investigator in the field of the lymphatic system. In a short life of nineteen years and seven months he accomplished a phenomenal amount of well planned investigation before he died of a dissection wound.

Charles was the eldest son of the physician scholar Erasmus Darwin (1731-1802) of Lichfield, Shropshire. It is from the father that we have the following description of his distinguished son. He was "accustomed to examine all natural objects with more attention than is usual: first by his senses simply; then by tools, which were his play-things—by this early use of his hands he gained accurate ideas of many of the qualities of bodies; and was thence afterwards enabled to acquire the knowledge of mechanics with ease and with accuracy; and the invention and improvement of machines was one of the first efforts of his ingenuity, and one of the first sources of his amusement.

"He had frequent opportunities in his early years of observing the various fossile productions in their native beds; and descended the mines of Derbyshire, and of some other county, with uncommon pleasure and observation. He collected with care the products of these countries; and examined them by such experiments, as he had been taught, or had discovered; hence he obtained not only distinct but indelible ideas of the properties of bodies, at the very time when he learnt the names of them; and thus the complicate science of chemistry became not only easy, but delightful to him."

After matriculation at Christ Church College, Oxford, in 1775 and spending a year there, he "sighed to be removed to the robuster exercises of the Medical Schools of Edinburgh." Thus in the early part of the year 1776 we find him vigorously engaged upon his medical studies under such professors as Robert Whytt in physiology, William Cullen, James Gregory, and Alexander Monro secundus, to whom we have elsewhere referred in this book. The Professor of the Theory of Medicine, Andrew Duncan, invited Charles Darwin to live in his home in Edinburgh and opened his wards at the Royal Infirmary to this comparatively young student soon after his arrival in Edinburgh. Charles Darwin's letters of this date foreshadow the discoveries to be made by this eager mind, and they radiate enthusiasm and high intellectual curiosity. Before graduating Darwin won the Gold Medal presented annually by the Aesculapian Society of Edinburgh for a dissertation on the characteristics of pus as distinct from mucus. His graduating essay or thesis was actually concerned with the lymphatics: "An Account of the Retrograde Motion from the Absorbent Vessels of Animal Bodies in Some Diseases." As his biographer, John Fulton, has said, "This was a more remarkable piece of work than the dissertation on pus and mucus, and it reflects the current teachings of Edinburgh concerning the relations of the lymphatics to dropsical conditions, and it also illustrates a very considerable independence of mind and a capacity to obtain evidence from well-conceived experiments." In addition Darwin wrote a remarkable essay of sixty-seven pages on "What are the established varieties of the pulse, their causes and uses in medicine." This was never published but was discovered by Fulton in the records of the Medical Society of London. This is one of his earliest pieces of work and showed that he knew a great deal about the background literature on studies of the heart and circulation. Among other things he describes the normal variation in the pulse that one finds in aging people, at rest, during exercise, eating, and sleeping. Thus, in three important fields, those of the body defences against infection, the lymphatic system, and the pulse, Darwin made quite remarkable investigations.

It was during such an investigation into hydrocephalus or "water on the brain" that the boy incurred a dissection wound which proved fatal in about two weeks' time. He developed a high fever with many haemorrhages into the tissues. So great was Dr. Andrew Duncan's affection for this student that he had him buried in the family vault in the Chapel of Ease of St. Cuthbert's at Edinburgh.

Darwin's diversified background learning was such that he would undoubtedly have been a great success in any calling. He has been overshadowed, of course, by his namesake Charles Robert Darwin but the combined roles of nature and nurture would seem to have lost none of their potency as one surveys the various members of this remarkable family. Darwin's father, Erasmus, was considered by some to be irascible, but at least he was energetic and saw to it that his son received a good general education. Erasmus waxed eloquent on some traditional methods in education when he wrote: "Ye classic schools! ye not only overcome the struggling efforts of genius and bind his Proteus-forms, till he speaks the language you require; but you then divert his attention from the nice comparison of things with each other, and from associating the ideas of causes and their effects; and amuse him with the looser analogies, the vain verbal allusions which constitute the ornaments of poetry and of oratory!" The little known Charles Darwin was indeed a remarkable exemplar of brilliant enquiry and insatiable curiosity flowering before the age of twenty.

→

PLATE 7

(a) Sir James Paget (1814-1899) from a portrait by George Richmond, 1867. From: Major, Ralph: *Classic Descriptions of Disease*, 1932. Courtesy of Charles C Thomas, Publisher.

(b) William Osler as a medical student at McGill University. Courtesy of Dr. W. W. Francis, The Osler Library.

(c) Ignaz Philipp Semmelweis (1818-1865). Courtesy of the Bettmann Archive, New York.

(d) Pecquet's student drawing of the lymphatic system in the dog. From: Stirling, W.: *Some Apostles of Physiology*, London, 1902.

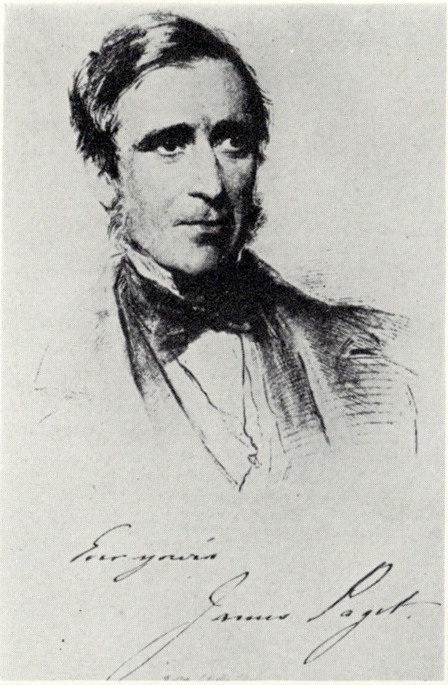

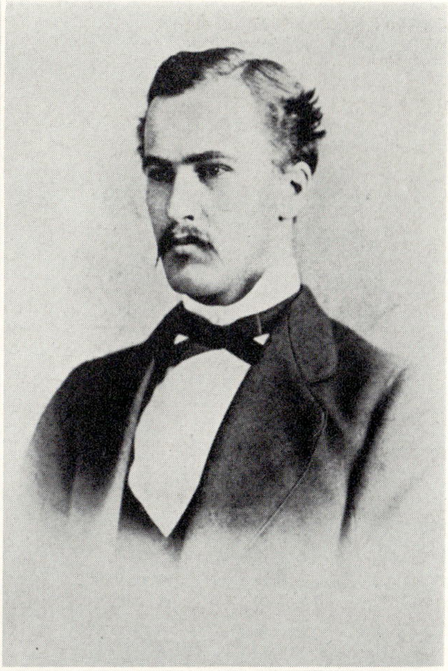

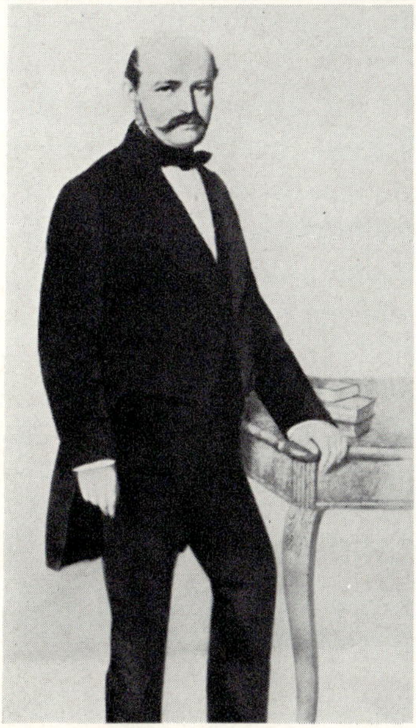

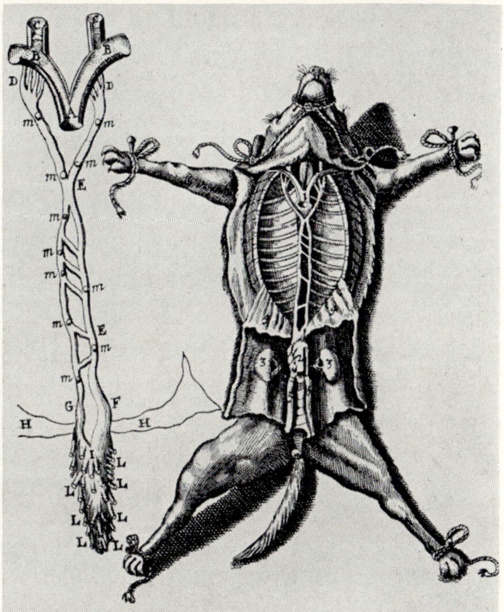

PECQUET'S FIGURE OF THE THORACIC DUCT IN THE DOG.

←

Chapter X

The Nervous System

THE BRAIN HAS known many kinds of investigators in its long history, isolated as it is in its bony enclosure, and insensitive itself to pain. The Edwin Smith papyrus, the oldest scientific document we have, shows that the Egyptians knew that an injury to one side of the brain affected the opposite side of the body. Gradually the idea evolved that there were localized areas on the surface of the brain controlling specific parts of the body. The present chapter will discuss the discoveries by medical students in the field of neurology, from the earliest attempts at cerebral localization to their contributions to the anatomy of the nerves, the pathological changes in the brain, the clinical diseases of humans, the physiology or functioning of the nervous system, and finally the student works of some pioneers in psychiatry.

CEREBRAL LOCALIZATION

The first of our student investigators in the field of brain structure was Francesco Gennari. He was born in 1750 in the village of Mataleto de Langhirano, near Parma, Italy. He studied medicine at Parma with the help of an annual bursary. His biographer, Marimo, states that Gennari was very openhanded with even this small subsidy and shared it with the indigent and with his gambling companions.

At the medical school in Parma, Gennari had the good fortune to fall under the spell of Michele Girardi, a most able teacher of pathology, and a pupil of Morgagni, the father of modern pathology. Girardi is known to medical historians as the editor of Santorini's works and as a pioneer in inoculation.

Girardi was himself possessed of an active mind and welcomed students who wished to investigate things for themselves. He provided a large number of cadavers for Gennari who was interested in the structure of the brain, and must have felt it worthwhile when Gennari, as an undergraduate, made his discovery of the white line in the visual area of the human brain.

To some this may seem an insignificant contribution to medical science, but its importance lies in the fact that it was the first discovery of that structural specialization of the cortex of the brain which today so occupies physiologists in search of functional correlates.

Gennari's little book, published in 1782, was dedicated to Count Giuseppe Camuti, Rector of the University of Parma, Court Physician and Professor of Chemistry. Its title ran: "De peculiari Structura cerebri nonnullisque eius morbis." It contained four copper plates, and was printed in Parma, probably by Bodoni. On page 72 he relates that on cutting the brain of a frozen cadaver, on February 2, 1776, he saw for the first time the line of "white matter," or "medulla," interposed between two layers of "gray matter," or "cortex," in the visual or occipital pole of the brain, posteriorly. A translation of his description follows:

"None of the anatomists I have come upon in reading have taught that, besides the cortical substance and the medulla, there exists in the brain another substance which I shall call the third substance of this viscus. If anyone has looked at the horizontal strata of the cortex of a brain dissected at the point where it conjoins with the medulla, he will have found a certain whitish substance ('subalbida'). This does not always present itself in exactly the same spot, appearing a little farther from or a little nearer to the medulla; it is however always observed with the same extension, with the same color, sometimes more abundant and sometimes more obscure; sometimes subtle, sometimes clearer; at points, difficult, at others it is easy to demonstrate. In a defect of a section especially if it is transected obliquely, this substance disappears; not only in single brains, but also in diverse parts of the same brain I have observed such variations, as if many times it reappeared in such points, *afterwards with a duplicate line* (Italics ours). Especially in the anterior parts or solely 'subobscure', it is possible to retrace it, but since it becomes denser to the posterior, I have come to the conclusion that its appearance can be more certainly obtained. In the internal part of the posterior lobe of the brain not far from the point in which it extends itself into the tentorium was where the substance of which I am speaking stretched in a line even whiter, but I have not observed it in any other place to be so evident.

"This line I first saw the 2nd February 1776 and having often followed it, it seemed to run finally to the ultimate substance of the hippocampus. For the rest I am ignorant to what purpose that substance may be formed, like so many others of which the use is still hidden, at any rate some of those who combat by the animal spirits, may perhaps draw such an argument for their existence, which in every time, even the hour in which I write, is much disputed. I exhort the anatomists in every way to enquire into this substance."

Little is known of the later life of Gennari, save that he published a case report on one of the hospital attendants and a "medical work" long since lost. It is known, however, from Verga's work on the brains of mental patients, published in Milan in 1896-97, that Gennari was greatly interested in the icicles which he found in the hollows or ventricles of the brain in frozen cadavers. He surmised, correctly, that since the frozen fluid was also interposed between the brain and its coverings, it served to cushion the brain against blows or sudden movements of the unyielding skull.

The date of Gennari's death is not known precisely, but it occurred some time before 1797, the year in which his teacher Girardi died. To Girardi, more than to anyone else, Gennari owed his fame, and he gracefully refers to his teacher in the preface to his book: "No one was superior to him and few have been his equal."

Fifty years after Gennari's discovery, a medical student in France, L. F. Bravais, was writing his thesis, "Recherches sur les symptômes et le traitment de l'épilepsie hémiplégique" in Paris. In this, for the first time, there was described a case with convulsions localized to a part only of the body. The French still refer to such a fit as a "crise Bravais-Jacksonienne."

Nine years later, in 1836, another French student, Marc Dax, wrote a thesis on his research on the brains of patients dying after the loss of speech (aphasia). He found that in right-handed aphasic patients the left hemisphere was selectively involved. Though he searched for a right-handed patient with a right cerebral lesion he never found one. This remarkable student wrote with a firm grip on the truth concerning aphasia. His thesis was never published, though copies of it existed in the Faculty of Medicine in Montpellier where he graduated, and where he had actually communicated the substance of his research to a medical congress in July, 1836. As Sir Geoffrey Jefferson has said, we must give "full credit to the prior observations of Marc Dax, who, before anyone else, observed that it was the left hemisphere that was usually found damaged in aphasics, a fact that did not dawn on Broca until he had seen Dax's posthumous but unpublished thesis."

Sir Henry Head (1861-1940) must be mentioned wherever aphasia and brain damage are discussed, so far-reaching were his studies. He came to this work well prepared, with a scholarly Quaker background, an honours B.A. degree in natural science from Cambridge, and two years of study in Prague and Halle before doing the clinical or hospital years of the medical course. In Prague he reputedly introduced soccer, while in Hering's laboratory in Halle he published two papers—one on the action potential of nerve and the second, in 1889, on the role of the vagus nerve in respiration. This was such a competent study that Head became widely known as an investigator. Upon qualifying with the M.B. degree in medicine at University College, London, Head wrote his M.D. thesis "On disturbance of sensation, with special reference to the pain of visceral disease," and this was of such high calibre that Hitzig insisted on its translation into German.

Head experimented on himself, cutting branches of the radial nerve in the arm to study changes in feeling in the skin affected.

His work on changes in sensation from brain injuries preceded World War I, and was greatly added to during that conflict. The speech difficulties associated with penetrating wounds of the head were studied in minutest detail and much of our descriptive terminology in this field today stems from Henry Head. As well as his medical works his verse was widely read. He died in 1940 after suffering, without complaint, from paralysis agitans for twenty years.

Very briefly we may refer to one of the keenest minds in the field of cerebral localization, the great French neurologist, Jean Martin Charcot (1825-1893). As a student, he contributed to our knowledge of arthritis and joint diseases. At the height of his powers Charcot was such a physician, teacher and artist that some would see him as the dividing line between the old neurology and the modern. This son of a carriage-builder shot like a comet across the sky, scattering light in such diverse fields as poliomyelitis, hysteria, epilepsy, cerebral function, multiple sclerosis, locomotor ataxia and the insensitive swollen joints which we now call "Charcot joints." Our principal interest here in Charcot is in his graduation thesis in medicine in 1848, entitled, "The affection described under the names of Primary Asthenic Gout, Nodosities of the Joints, and the Primary Form of Chronic Articular Rheumatism." It was in this student work that he sorted out for the first time the waste-basket classification of joint disease. It reflects his systematic approach to the mélange of arthritic problems which he saw lumped together in the wards of the Salpêtriere. This sense of discernment is to be seen over and over again in the work of French physicians, whose clinical observations set off a chain-reaction in basic research—Charcot, Claude Bernard, and Broca being pre-eminent in this regard.

When it became possible to speak of specific areas of the brain being connected with definite functions of the human body, neurologists began to wonder if special microscopic structures were involved. For instance, were motor areas on the surface of the brain similar in composition to sensory areas?

One of the first to provide answers to this problem was Constantin von Economo (1876-1931), a restless son of aristocratic Greek parents. He first studied engineering, to please his father, and was, after two years, allowed to proceed to medicine upon which his mind had been set since the age of fourteen when he had read Lombroso's book, *Genius and Insanity*. Baron von Economo graduated in medicine in Vienna after writing an undergraduate paper on the pituitary gland in birds. His early endocrinological interests gave way to those for which he is famous today—the parcelation of the surface of the human brain according to its microscopic structure. He pursued this interest from 1912 until his death in 1931, with frequent interruptions, usually concerned with aeronautics! In 1908 he had learned to fly aeroplanes, and gave up balloons. He fought as a pilot in the First World War and became prominent in an early movement to get airports built in major cities. His life was nothing if not varied.

Important as it was to appreciate the relation between structure and function in the cerebral cortex, it was still more important to develop the technical methods for showing up the precise microscopic anatomy of the various brain areas. Rudolph Berlin, as a twenty-five year old medical student at Erlangen, in 1858, reported on his researches in this field in his graduation dissertation of twenty-seven pages. He illustrated his little work with two plates, and his designation of the cells which he stained, as pyramidal, spindle and granular, we still use daily.

We should not leave this matter of localization of function in the brain without a reference to the pioneering work done by Niclas and Spurzheim as student assistants to the father of phrenology, Franz Joseph Gall (1757-1828). Though Gall operated on fantastic assumptions at times, his labors in Paris undoubtedly advanced the problems to the stage where Bravais, Dax and Broca could help to solve them.

NEUROANATOMISTS

The work of gross anatomists has been covered generally in Chapter II. However, there remain for consideration here some student contributors whose work lay largely in the nervous system, such as the Meckels and R. B. Hirsch. Johann Friedrich Meckel (1724-1774) established a line of Prussian anatomists—father, son and two grandsons. He was born at Wetzlar and graduated in medicine in 1748 with a dissertation on the anatomy and physiology of the "fifth pair of nerves from the brain." In this he described for the first time the spheno-palatine ganglion, since called Meckel's ganglion, lodged, as the name implies, in the bony cavities above the palate and below the base of the skull.

In the same year Meckel described the submaxillary ganglion which lies at the angle of the human jawbone and is protected by it. These studies were soon extended to the innervation of the face. Three years after graduation he was made a professor in Berlin where he taught botany, anatomy and obstetrics. In fact he was the first physician to give instruction in midwifery at La Charité Hospital there.

When J. F. Meckel's son, Phillip Friedrich Theodor Meckel (1756-1803) graduated in medicine in Strasbourg in 1777 he wrote an important dissertation on the labyrinth of the internal ear. He became professor of anatomy at Halle two years later, and was eventually obstetrician to the Russian court. His two sons were also distinguished anatomists, particularly Johann Friedrich (1781-1833) who has been called "the German Cuvier," so eminent was he in the fields of comparative anatomy and pathology. From 1821 to 1830 he wrote his great system of comparative anatomy which demonstrated the recapitulation of earlier attributes at some stage of the development of higher animals.

One of Meckel's most distinguished pupils was Alexander Monro, Secundus (1733-1817), son of the Professor of Anatomy at Edinburgh, and father of Alexander Monro, Tertius, who completed the 128-year dynasty in which the three Monros occupied the Chair of Anatomy at Edinburgh. Monro, Secundus, studied in London under William Hunter, the distinguished older brother of John and the brilliant teacher of the Great Windmill Street School of anatomy in London. Of this period Monro has written:

> So far back as 1753, soon after I began the study of Anatomy, I discovered that the Lateral Ventricles of the Human Brain communicated with each other, *and*, at the same place with the Middle or Third Ventricle of the Brain: And, as a passage from the Third Ventricle to the Fourth is universally known, it followed, that what are called the Four Ventricles of the Brain, are in reality different parts of one cavity.

The Foramen of Monro, thus described, has become familiar to all medical students since, which is quite a number! Monro himself lectured to forty thousand of them in his fifty years as Professor at Edinburgh—a post which he assumed at the age of twenty-five. He was a brilliant teacher of anatomy and the leading physician of his time in Edinburgh. He was a fearless controversialist and as a young man crossed swords with William Hunter over priority in discovery of the function of the lymphatics. Monro had done considerable undergraduate work on these vessels and actually wrote his thesis on them, "De Venis Lymphaticus Valvulosis," in Berlin, at the age of twenty-four. We know from a letter of Joseph Black, the chemist, that Monro had been working on the vessels at the age of twenty-two, and had, by a very ingenious method, shown that the lymphatics "are a distinct system of vessels, having no immediate connection with the arteries and veins, but arising, in small branches, from all the cavities and cells in the body, into which fluids are thrown; and that their use is to absorb the whole, or the thinner parts of these fluids, and restore them to the mass of circulating humours." By injecting fluids into arteries against the direction of the stream of blood he was able to show, in the lungs, that the foreign matter thus injected was taken up by the thin lymphatic vessels and transported away by them.

Monro's other original contributions were concerned (a) with the little cushions or bursae underlying some muscles, the seat of the common disease "bursitis," and (b) with the comparative anatomy and physiology of fishes.

Domenico Cotugno (1736-1822)

Any biographical note on this remarkable man might be entitled "The father of Sciatica" or "From radishes to Rectorship." Thanks to the diligent researches of Dr. Henry Viets, the Boston historian and neurologist, Cotugno's fascinating life has been rescued from oblivion, and to him all students of history are genuinely indebted.

Cotugno was born on the southern Adriatic coast of Italy and grew up with his brothers in very humble circumstances. The feudal lord in this part of Italy, the Duca d'Andria, sponsored his entrance into the University of Naples. It was Cotugno's good fortune to encounter there a wise professor of philosophy, Antonio Genovesi, who told him: "If you have an original idea write it down and put it among your papers; after some time read it, and perhaps a second idea will come to mind in a similar manner to the first. Add this to the original thought and later re-read them both. A third and fourth idea may be created and perhaps a complete work will be the result of the first idea." The student took this advice so literally that he wrote three medical books by the time he was aged thirty-two.

Cotugno began his medical training at seventeen and within his first year began to study sciatica and its causes. His financial situation was pitiful. He asked for and was given some sort of work in the Ospedali degli Incurabili; he was classed there at age nineteen as "resident physician." This more fittingly described his duties than his rewards, and he lived on radishes and bread until he suffered an haemoptysis, possibly tuberculous in origin. The hospital authorities thereupon provided him with a better room and a much better diet.

Before long he was tutoring surgical students in anatomy, a subject which he liked so much that he made independent dissections on hundreds of dogs, rabbits, birds, rats and humans. He became interested in the secrets locked securely in the petrous portion of the temporal bone of the skull. Subsequent generations have probably wished that Cotugno had never uncovered the series of traps which this intricate area holds for the student being examined in anatomy. However, Cotugno was not being examined, he was examining and he found a veritable gold mine. He found that there were two nerves to the ear, one for hearing and one for balance. He found the semi-circular canals, connected with the latter, to contain a clear liquid, the better to remind us of our position in space. He thought that the spiral cochlea, or shell-like organ of hearing, had represented on its two-and-one-half turns the necessary structures for recording and distinguishing pitch. This, we should remember, was a century before Helmholtz proved it so in detail. This investigation which he began as a third year student was published in Naples in 1761 as *De Aquaeductibus Auris Internae—Anatomica Dissertatio*.

His research on sciatica and the cerebrospinal fluid was continued for ten years before he published on it at the age of twenty-eight. The whole treatise is a masterpiece of exposition. He begins by differentiating from sciatica all those afflictions which superficially resemble it, such as arthritis, sacroiliac disease and tuberculous affections of the spine.

In describing the origin of the sciatic nerve from the lower segments of the spinal cord he introduces the subject of the clear liquid which surrounds the cord and which is contained by the meninges. He notes that it resembles the fluid found in the pericardial sac about the heart, or that found in the hollows of the brain and the semicircular canals of the ear, and "in other cavities of the body impervious to the air."

Occasionally, he says, the fluid is yellow, but it is invariably red and opaque in the case of a foetus strangled in a difficult labor. He thinks the liquid is manufactured by the choroid plexus in the hollows of the brain and is re-absorbed over the surface of the brain, as we do today. He thought the liquid "to be in a continual state of renovation," which view is borne out by "modern" studies using radio-active isotopes.

The causes of sciatica were difficult to ascertain but, in cadavers, he forced air and quicksilver along the sciatic nerve elements peripherally in search of blocks, compressions and other affections. He knew that the lifting of heavy weights could lead to sciatica. His general conclusion was that the cerebrospinal fluid itself caused the pain, and in support of this he was able to demonstrate "dropsy of the nerve" in known cases.

Valsalva is said to have mentioned the spinal fluid in 1692, noting that it resembled the fluid within the joints of the limbs. In order to be sure that the fluid did not arise post-mortem, Cotugno experimented on sea tortoises and found it present during life. He showed that there were times when the fluid was coagulated. This is of interest in view of the fact that Cotugno was the first to show that albumen in the urine could be coagulated by heat. His other discoveries include the nasopalatine nerve, according to Castiglioni, and it is recorded that in 1784 "while dissecting a mouse, he observed, imperfectly, animal electricity."

It is little wonder that Cotugno became Professor of Anatomy at Naples, and was known to the great pathologist Morgagni of Padua. As the wheel came full circle the erstwhile "resident physician" aged nineteen became the leading physician of Naples, Chief of Service at the "Incurabili," Dean of Medicine of the University, and finally Rector. Before he died he headed the Royal Academy of Sciences. He started the preventive movement in the field of tuberculosis in Naples.

Throughout his long and constructive professional life he maintained a dispensary for poor patients in his home. In gratitude for shelter when he most needed it, and for the opportunity to study, he left his fortune to the Hospital for Incurables. His life was determined in large measure by the hospital to which he turned as a penniless youth, in a manner reminiscent of John Shaw Billings' life. Small hospitals will probably always have souls, and the educational opportunity which they present to the enquiring mind is as limitless as it is unique. If the walls of such hospitals could speak they would tell of a camaraderie, unknown to oft-vacant lecture halls, but regnant in the wards and corridors where human beings are born, are cared for and die—where from midnight to midnight, century after century, a living river flows. Perhaps the incurable patients in the wards of his little hospital were in Cotugno's mind when he wrote: "Medicine does not have masters; it has but one teacher, Nature."

It is pleasant to be able to record that one student, R. B. Hirsch, in his graduation thesis in Vienna in 1765, memorialized his teacher Johann Ludwig Gasser in naming the great sensory ganglion which supplies the face, the Gasserian ganglion. One is reminded of Christopher Wren's famous drawing of the arterial circle at the base of the brain which, it is said, he named "the circle of Willis," after his teacher at Oxford. While on the subject of Willis, it might be added that the method of naming and numbering the cranial nerves—those to the eyes, ears, tongue and so on, which he devised, was eventually replaced by an improved system which originated with a German medical student. In 1778 Samuel Thomas von Soemmering presented this new classification of the cranial nerves in his graduation thesis. He became a remarkable physician, a disciple of Jenner, a contributor to physics and to the early work which preceded the electric telegraph. Independently he described the "white line of Gennari" in the gray matter of the human brain. He wrote on sunspots and on fossils. Thirteen years after graduation he described the disease of developing structures known as achondroplasia. The classical description of this condition, however, was to await the talented medical student, M. H. Romberg (1795-1873), whose graduation thesis, "On Congenital Rickets," in Berlin in 1817 embodied a most thorough study. Every student knows Romberg's name in connection with the loss of the erect posture with the eyes closed in certain ataxic disorders.

Before completing our section on anatomists of the nervous system we must chronicle briefly the career of one whose life span covered almost a century—a century in which the microscope came to displace the scalpel in laboratories dedicated to research. Rudolf Albert von Kölliker (1817-1905) was one of the truly noble creations of Nature—a Swiss mountaineer with the presence and resourcefulness of a guide—approachable, the friend of young men struggling uphill, and a great teacher.

As a medical student in Bonn and Berlin, he spent his summers in Heligoland in zoological investigations. They culminated, two years before he graduated in medicine, in a publication on the sexual physiology of the invertebrates. From 1847 to 1902—a period of fifty-five years—he served as head of the Institute of Comparative Anatomy, Microscopy and Embryology at Wurzburg—retiring at the age of 85 years! Gerhardt von Bonin relates that Kölliker in the last eight years of his life published twenty papers.

Kölliker was one of the important forerunners of "the neurone theory" and years before it was popularized wrote: "All nerve cells must have essentially the same function and their functional dignity depends solely upon the different extraneous stimuli which might impinge upon them or upon the many possibilities of answers to a stimulus." (von Bonin) He championed the work of the unknown stranger from Spain—Ramón y Cajal—at a meeting of the German Anatomical Society held under his chairmanship in Berlin in 1889.

He stands as one of the most benevolent and human figures in the history of neurology. His contributions were truly great, his meticulous textbooks milestones in themselves, and his encouragement of young scientists a monument to his memory.

Robert Remak (1815-1865)

Polish patriots living within the borders of Germany have never led an easy life. Robert Remak was born in Posen soon after its incorporation into Prussia following Napoleon's defeat. Remak was the son of a local merchant and attended the Gymnasium in Posen. On his graduation there his schoolmaster wrote of him: "Diligence, attendance and conduct must be regarded as exemplary. Progress in all subjects was excellent so that I am able to certify with good conscience I never before had such an excellent pupil in my class." At the age of eighteen he earned a place in the Medical Faculty of the University of Berlin where he soon came under the spell of the outstanding German physiologist of the century, Johannes Müller. With Müller's personal microscope Remak embarked on a study of the finest nerve fibres in the body, a study which he published three years later, and incorporated in his graduation thesis in 1838. Such was the worth of his contribution to knowledge that we still refer to these nerve fibres as "Remak's fibres."

His investigation showed that the principal structure in any nerve fibre was the central core of conducting material known as the "axis cylinder," and that this material was continuous with the interior of the single nerve cell from which it originated. He showed, moreover, that there was a preponderance of those non-medullated or non-insulated fibres in what he called "the organic nervous system"—which today we speak of as "the autonomic nervous system" because it regulates digestion, blood pressure and many vital functions while we sleep. Remak's vertebrate conclusions were confirmed in the invertebrate nervous system five years later by another medical student, Helmholtz.

Remak's 42-page thesis was entitled: "Observationes anatomicae et microscopicae de systematis nervosi structura," and began with a quotation from Francis Bacon, "Neither manual work alone nor imagination unchecked by facts is worth very much." His text and drawings attracted the favorable notice of Alexander von Humboldt, the naturalist and explorer.

From his graduation in 1838 to his death twenty-seven years later Remak's contributions to knowledge simply poured out as if from an inexhaustible fountain. His interests ranged from retinal physiology to the nervous structures of the tongue, the larynx, pharynx, bronchi and lungs, to the liver and its prolific nerve supply, to red blood cells, ossification, involuntary muscle, the secretion of glands and to localization on the brain of visceral functions of the body.

After lecturing in his apartment for twenty years he was invited to lecture in the University of Berlin. His importance in the development of "the cell theory" is poorly recognized still. He supplied the theory, "omnis cellula et cellula," which was to make Virchow famous. Like John Hunter, he worked on inflammation and the blocking of blood vessels, and extended his researches to the stimulation of blood regeneration by the bleeding of horses, to the absorbing structures of the intestine, to the inflammation of the lining membrane of the lungs in pneumonia and to the single muscle cell which he showed to be the unit of all our muscles. He first described the disorder known as pulsus paradoxus in 1844. He pioneered in the field of the development of the embryo and wrote of the germinal layers from which the tissues of the body are selectively developed. His student researches, however, proved to be the central core around which his other fundamental contributions to neurology were grouped. His stature in the history of this subject is likely to grow larger as time goes on.

Theodore Billroth (1829-1894)

Theodore Billroth is well-known as one of Germany's greatest surgeons of the nineteenth century. As an undergraduate he and Meissner assisted Professor Wagner in physiological research and accompanied him to Trieste in 1851 where they did a microscopic study of the nerves of the electric ray. It was as a result of this apprenticeship at the microscope, similar to that of the young Joseph Lister, that Billroth turned to experimental pathology and wrote his graduation thesis in 1852 on, "The nature and cause of a pulmonary affection which arises from cutting the vagus nerve," at the age of twenty-three. His first teaching post was in pathological anatomy and from a sound background in the post-mortem and microscopic observation of diseased tissues he went on to surgery. He was a teacher who trained teachers, among them the brilliant abdominal surgeon, Mikulicz, and the versatile Kocher of Switzerland. His textbooks passed through eight editions during his life-time and his name is still a "household" word in surgery. In the field of music he is well-known, as a close friend of Brahms who dedicated various works to him, and as the author of a most interesting work, "Psycho-physiological aphorisms on music."

We come now to that enigmatic dynamo, Sir Victor Horsley (1857-1916)—an anatomist as an undergraduate. The third child born to John Callcott Horsley, R.A., and his wife was named Victor at the request of Queen Victoria. He was born in Kensington into a family of unusual gifts. His mother was descended from a long line of artists and surgeons, and was herself raised in France. His father came of a family of musicians and artists. He combined a hot temper with generosity and, above all, activity. On occasion he found it necessary to write to *The Times* cautioning against the dangers of modernity.

A year after Victor's birth the family moved to Cranbrook in Kent, and the formative fifteen years of his life were spent in this country setting. He became an observer of everything in Nature, and his childhood letters are remarkable for the detail with which he describes the birds' nests, silkworms, boats and people that he encountered. At the age of fifteen he decided that he would study medicine, and at once began to dissect birds, and to work with the microscope. Like Osler, he ground his own sections of bone for observation.

In January, 1874, he matriculated at the University of London. He attended lectures at University College and was tutored by Philip Magnus. In July, 1875, he passed his preliminary science examinations and was awarded the Gold Medal in Anatomy. From this time until July, 1878, he concentrated on physiology under Burdon Sanderson and Shafer. His classmates numbered among them C. E. Beevor, Francis Gotch, F. W. Mott and Dudley Buxton.

Horsley's biographer, Stephen Paget, relates that as an undergraduate Horsley gave two papers to the Students' Medical Society of University College embodying his own researches. The first, given during the session of 1875-76, was entitled, "On the endings of the tendons in the rat's tail." The other, presented a year later, was, "On the terminations of muscular fibres; and a note on the structure of intervertebral discs." This long and painstaking paper, based upon excellent microscopic work, was awarded a prize by the Students' Society, which also elected him as President for the year.

After completing the 1876-77 term with further distinctions and medals, Horsley travelled in Germany for four weeks. His diary for the month covers 120 pages. He carried a letter of introduction from Burdon Sanderson and visited a number of laboratories. His criticisms of some laboratories were very cryptic. He saw, however, in Strasbourg, some of the dogs on whose brain Professor Goltz had operated, and this made a lasting impression on him.

At "The Club" in University College, Horsley gave a well illustrated lecture on Reformed Dress for Women. He favored "trousers to the ankle" and a "very full frock-coat buttoned up to the throat." He also took up the anti-alcohol, anti-tobacco crusade, which was later to waste so much of his energy in fruitless political struggles.

As Horsley progressed into the clinical part of his course, his interests turned to pathological anatomy, in which he won the Filliter Exhibition. His regular attendance at operations soon overcame his fainting tendencies. His artistic abilities were often called upon by his Chiefs, and in 1879 we find him drawing the relations of the spinal nerves to the vertebral column for a lecture by Gowers. While clerking for Bastian, Horsley drew two plates for his book, *The Brain as an Organ of the Mind.* In the April issue of *Brain* in 1880, Horsley published, with Bastian, a very important paper, "Arrest of development in the left upper limb in association with an extremely small right ascending parietal convolution." The drawings were by Horsley.

It was clear in what direction he was heading, as his association with the neurologists Gowers and Bastian developed. Another of his teachers was Rickman Godlee, who was the first surgeon to remove a brain tumor which had been localized pre-operatively through a study of the attendant clinical signs and symptoms.

While a student, Horsley also carried on bacteriological work with F. W. Mott, although their paper was not published until 1882.

In November of 1880, Horsley took his M.R.C.S., which allowed him to practise, and in 1881 he completed his University of London M.B., B.S., winning the Gold Medal in Surgery. He lost no time in taking off for the Continent for a breathing spell, and visited the laboratory of the noted pathologist Cohnheim in Leipzig. On his return to London, Horsley once more took up bacteriology, and was interested in the demonstration of the tubercle bacillus under the microscope. He worked on the transplanting of tumors from man to cats, and from rats to rabbits. His clinical observation of a sick mouse, which he encountered in a railway cut at Wimbledon, led him to examine its blood, which he found to be alive with trypanosomes.

The incessant activity inherited from his father was manifest at all times, but between drawing illustrations for the ninth edition of Quain's Anatomy and reading a paper on December 13, 1883, to the Physiological Society, "On four cases of injury to the brain; illustrating the position of the motor centres," Horsley found time to take his F.R.C.S. John Marshall prevailed on him to illustrate the Bradshaw Lecture for him, "On the operation of nerve stretching for the relief or cure of pain."

From 1884 to 1890, Horsley served as Professor Superintendent of the Brown Institution, that singular research centre which can boast among its one-time chiefs, Burdon Sanderson, Greenfield, Roy, Sherrington, Rose Bradford and Brodie. It was established in 1871 by the will of Mr. Thomas Brown of Dublin, "for the founding, establishing and upholding of an Institution for investigating, studying, and without charge beyond immediate expenses, endeavouring to cure maladies, distempers, and injuries, (which) any quadrupeds or birds useful to man may be found subject to." The University of London was "to control the number and cases of diseased or injured animals to be taken charge of, and to decide about the purchase of diseased or injured animals or their carcases for the promotion of science."

Horsley's work at the Brown Institution was along three main lines. First was his study of the localization of function in the brains of animals, with related studies on the pathology of epilepsy and of chorea in dogs. Second was his pioneer work on thyroid gland deficiencies as related to myxoedema and cretinism. The third segment of his investigations was on means of protection against rabies.

As neurosurgical practice and political campaigning came to absorb more of Horsley's time and energy so did his scientific publications decrease in frequency. In 1908, he presented to the Royal Society a very interesting report on the brain of Mr. Charles Babbage, F.R.S., who invented intricate mechanical calculators a century ago, and who proposed, in vain, a design for a reflecting ophthalmoscope to Wharton Jones in 1845. In 1908, also, Horsley and R. H. Clarke published an account of their now famous stereotaxic apparatus for the exact placing of electrodes at predetermined points within the brain.

In 1911, Horsley received a prize from the Société de Chirurgie of Paris for having made the greatest contribution to the advancement of surgery in the preceding ten years. He also received a white kangaroo from a grateful patient in Australia.

Horsley, the father of neurosurgery, had opened the door on the most difficult of all surgical specialties. He had shown that it was possible to learn something about the human brain while attempting surgically to cure some of its grosser maladies. While he did this, and made his own artistic drawings, and labored too in opening the field of endocrinology, so a younger man across the Atlantic—Harvey Cushing—persevered, refined neurosurgical techniques, transfused his cases with blood, skillfully sketched his operative fields and, not least of all, broke down the barriers of ignorance that surrounded the functions of the pituitary gland. Both men soon became enmeshed in the war of 1914, Cushing first having to fight a political battle on Boston Common, and Horsley first having to condemn the rotten heart of Europe. On August 25, 1914, Horsley wrote to a colleague: "The situation is exactly what you would expect from the aristocrats who rule Europe. Austria trying to smash Servia; Germany coolly smashing Belgium. Burglary and murder arranged in the name of God by rulers and nobles. And all the while the people who are starved, tortured and killed have not had a single voice in the matter."

"I dreamed of you last night—operating on Hughlings Jackson. The great principle you said, in cerebral surgery, was to create a commotion by which the association paths were restored. You took off the scalp, like a p.m. incision—made a big hole over the cerebellum and put in a Christ Church (Oxford)-whipped cream wooden instrument and rotated it rapidly. Then you put back the bone and sewed him up. You said he would never have a fit again. I said solemnly, 'I'm not surprised.' Hughlings Jackson seemed very comfortable after the operation and bought three oranges from a small Neopolitan who strayed into the Queen Square amphitheatre!"

—W. Osler to Harvey Cushing (1909).

Horsley was among the first to volunteer for service and was despatched eventually to Egypt. He then served in Gallipoli, India and finally in Mesopotamia. His letters were full of delightful little sketches of people and things seen. His student interest in archeology was revived. But he was restless and heedless of danger. He succumbed to heat stroke on July 16, 1916, after walking miles at midday to attend an ailing colleague.

Horsley willed his skull and brain to the Neurological Society of London, and the rest of his body to University College, London, for the preparation of anatomical specimens for the museum. This was typical of his complex, inflexible and generous nature.

In a busy lifetime with many peripheral interests Horsley managed to contribute 125 papers to the medical literature. He slaved all his life for medicine, as a student, as a researcher and teacher, as a surgeon, and finally as a soldier. We can understand what he meant when at age fifty-eight he said good-bye to his wife in Egypt: "Don't worry about me; I don't matter; I can't live forever; it's the young that matter."

Student contributors in the field of psychiatry may have been few but they became the pillars of this important branch of medicine. J. E. D. Esquirol (1772-1840), the favorite pupil of Pinel the reformer, wrote his graduation thesis in 1805 on "The emotions considered as causes, symptoms and curative means in the field of mental illness." The tide was just beginning to turn in the vast sea of torture and abuse to which mental patients had been subjected. The lashing and chaining of patients and the "non-injurious torture" prescribed by Reil among others—such as shooting off cannon and ducking patients in water—was being replaced by Pinel's humane approach. If it took courage on Pinel's part to strike the chains from the incarcerated patients, it probably took more courage on the part of the medical student Esquirol to say that this controversial treatment was right and had a sound scientific basis.

Esquirol's later life bore out the promise of his early years. He introduced many things into psychiatry: the use of the statistical method in mental disease; the term "hallucination" as we understand it today; and a saner outlook on responsibility before the law of mentally sick people. Like his teacher, Pinel, he was an innovator in a long-ignored field of medicine. In turn, his own students, such as Baillarger, carried the torch, and campaigned for the rehabilitation of patients discharged from mental hospitals —a labor of love still crying out to be done effectively.

The versatile August Forel (1848-1931) is remembered the world over for his studies on ants and their social behavior. Like so many Swiss physicians he was a biologist with a broad base of experience and manifold interests. At the age of seven, on the shores of Lake Geneva, he became enamoured of ants, and wherever he went, in his schooling, he kept learning their lore. When he entered medical school in Zurich in 1866 he was already writing papers on ants, and when, thirty-two years later, he retired from his chair of psychiatry there, he was still writing about them.

As a medical student Forel came under the spell of the gifted von Gudden—a pioneer in neuroanatomy and psychiatry, later to be drowned by his patient, Ludwig II, the mad king of Bavaria. Forel's doctoral thesis was begun in 1871 under the famous anatomist Meynert. It was a contribution to the structure of the mammalian thalamus and its role in vision. Meynert disagreed with some of his student's conclusions, but he had the grace, nevertheless, to have it published in the Proceedings of the Vienna Academy of Sciences.

Fortunately for science Forel failed in a competition for a local health officer's appointment, though he bitterly resented the petty medical politics which entered into the selection. Within eight years he was made Professor of Psychiatry at Zurich succeeding that pioneer in electrical stimulation of the brain, Eduard Hitzig. Forel was also made Director of the Burgholzi Asylum. He clearly enunciated the "neurone theory" in 1877 quite independently. With Oskar Vogt he founded the famous *Journal für Psychologie und Neurologie.* His crusading pen was stilled temporarily at the age of sixty-four by a stroke, but he learned to write with his left hand and continued on until his death at the age of eighty-three.

Sigmund Freud (1856-1939)

It may come as a sobering thought to some to learn that one of the most controversial figures in the history of medicine and thought, Sigmund Freud, was a student investigator in anatomy. Freud did not emerge from some sort of penny-in-the-slot machine with psychoanalysis on his lips, at the turn of the century. Rather he came from the exacting discipline of the neuro-anatomical laboratory and from the hard realities of speech disorders and cerebral palsy in the neurological clinic.

Freud was born in Freiberg in Moravia, and from the age of four lived in Vienna. In grammar school he was a consistently good student and developed broad cultural interests. He was early conscious of the Darwinian theories which were then breaking on the world.

Despite the fact that his family lived in straitened circumstances, Freud nevertheless embarked on an education for the medical profession, although at one time he was on the verge of studying law. However, his reading of Goethe's essay *Die Nature* determined him on a medical career.

Freud entered the University of Vienna in 1873. In 1876 he commenced to work, as a student, in Ernst Brucke's Laboratory of Physiology, and continued almost uninterruptedly until 1882. He graduated with his M.D. degree in 1881, aged 25. The first study set him by Brucke concerned a larval form of the early vertebrate, Petromyzon. One might speculate that this was the beginning of Freud's thinking concerning phylogeny and levels of development and of function within the nervous system.

On January 4, 1877, Brucke communicated Freud's first paper to the Vienna Academy of Science. It was entitled "Spinal Ganglia and the Spinal Cord of Petromyzon" and was later printed, being twelve pages in length and accompanied by a color plate. In 1878 the study was elaborated into one of eighty pages and four plates. He clearly showed the derivation of unipolar posterior root ganglion cells from bipolar sensory cells in this species. It might be noted here that Freud was no newcomer to the field of comparative neurology, having spent the summer of 1876 with Professor Clause, of the Institute of Comparative Anatomy in Vienna, at the Zoological Station at Trieste.

Freud was one of the lesser forerunners of the "neurone theory" as it came to be called in Germany. In the summers of 1879 and 1880 he worked on the nervous system of the fresh water crab

"At Paris you always can advance yourself by work and enthusiasm. You don't need any 'relations.' You are the product of your work."

—Joseph Jules Dejerine (1849-1917).

"Understanding is the reward, not of the gifts of genius, but of the expenditure of effort."

—Sigmund Freud.

and emphasized the finely neurofibrillar structure of their axones. He was impressed also by the similarity of the pattern of the nervous system in invertebrates and vertebrates.

From Brucke's laboratory, also, Freud published his papers on the tracts and nuclei within the medulla oblongata. At about the same period (1880) he translated into German John Stuart Mill's book, *The Emancipation of Women.* Freud's co-workers in Brucke's laboratory had equally broad interests and published on such subjects as: collateral innervation, the origin of cell nuclei, corneal innervation, the conception of movement and space, and "the nature of the psychical process."

Freud graduated in 1881, and in 1882, on Brucke's advice, embarked on a clinical training as his only hope of earning a living. While on the neurological service of the Allgemeines Krankenhaus in Vienna, Freud found time to carry on some neuropathological studies in Meynert's laboratory. One of these was on the use of gold salts in the staining of the axones of nerve cells as a means of tracing fibre tracts in the nervous system.

His papers thereafter show an increasing preoccupation with clinical neuropathological matters, such as cerebral and basal ganglion lesions in a case of scurvy, muscular atrophy associated with syringomyelia, and acute mutiple neuritis. With Meynert he wrote a paper on the acoustic nucleus and the interolivary tract.

In 1884 Freud received a supply of cocaine from the Merck Company and carried on many experiments with it. These are detailed in a small book which he produced on the subject. He told his ophthalmological colleagues Konigstein and Carl Koller of its potential value in anaesthetizing the eye. Returning from a vacation he found that Koller had publicly demonstrated this effect in animals. Freud tested the effect of cocaine on human endurance, and with a dynamometer was able to show that the effect was not subjective only.

In 1885 Freud was awarded a travelling fellowship in neuropathology which took him to Paris. There he worked with Darkschewitsch on the connections of the inferior peduncle of the cerebellum with the posterior columns of the spinal cord, which had not been understood previously. Freud's apprenticeship in comparative neurology came to his assistance when he developed the thesis of the homology of the sensory nuclei in the medulla oblongata with the posterior roots of the spinal cord at a lower level.

Despite all this, however, Charcot's Clinic became the outstanding interest of Freud in Paris. At the Salpêtrière he heard the great clinician say that he wished his lectures might be translated into German. Freud offered to carry out this onerous work and was soon admitted to the inner circle. The chief interests of Charcot at that moment were hypnosis, suggestion and hysterical paralyses and contractures. Freud suggested that study might be made of organic paralyses as compared with those of an hysterical nature, which always conformed to the patient's view of such phenomena. However, as Freud remarks in his Autobiography, Charcot "took no special interest in penetrating more deeply into the psychology of the neuroses."

Returning from Paris in 1886, Freud spent some time in Berlin at paediatric clinics, with a view to future collaboration with Kassowitz in Vienna. Actually some of Freud's best clinical studies came out of Kassowitz's institute, on "The Cerebral Palsies of Children."

On returning to Vienna, Freud gave to the Society of Medicine an account of his tenure of the travelling fellowship in neuropathology. As he recounted the things which he had seen and learned in Paris he was given the "prophet without honour" reception reserved for returning post-graduate fellows in the medical profession. His attempts to get access to patients to prove what he was talking about were as ineffectual as those of Semmelweis, forty years earlier, in the same hospital, who had been denied access even to his own clinical records. The laboratory of anatomy was closed to Freud, and he was allowed no place in which to lecture.

Locked out, therefore, Freud began medical practice with what he called "the crowds of neurotics whose number seemed further multiplied by the manner in which they hurried, with their troubles unsolved, from one physician to another." Using electrical machines and hypnotism he waded into the totally uncharted sea of psychotherapy. He soon gave up the electrotherapy and began to move towards the use of suggestion in therapy. As he later wrote: "Psychoanalysis is the administrator of the estate left by hypnotism."

He travelled to Nancy to observe Liébault and Bernheim, as he says, "working among the poor women and children of the labouring classes, . . . and I received the profoundest impression of the possibility that there could be powerful mental processes which nevertheless remained hidden from the consciousness of men."

In 1891 Freud published his work on "Aphasia" and showed that he had grasped the significance of the great generalizations being propounded in England by Hughlings Jackson in this field, such as "the dissolution of function." This was followed, in 1893, by a monograph of 168 pages on cerebral diplegia, a work which drew the praise of Pierre Marie. In the same year Freud, in company with his old colleague from Brucke's laboratory, Josef Breuer, wrote "On the Psychic Mechanisms of Hysterical Phenomena."

With this publication and with his translation of Bernheim's 414-page book on suggestion, Freud started out upon his second "ink-pot career," though this one completely overshadowed his first in volume of writing. As if Freud had not written enough on psychoanalysis, a band of interpreters has arisen, and at the hands of some of these Freud has suffered. The importance of what he had to say is too great to allow it to be drowned in the currently fashionable semantic torrent, and for that reason a brief and clear summary by Franz Alexander is quoted in part: "Freud's main accomplishments were to demonstrate that man's personality, normal or morbid, is shaped by life experiences; that among these experiences early childhood experiences are of overwhelming significance and, above all, that behind a layer of civilized veneer man harbors in his unconscious mind an asocial nucleus with destructive impulses directed against others and himself. He discovered a method by which this asocial core of the personality can be explored in spite of man's natural tendency to hide it from himself and others. Freud called this tendency repression, and the method by which repressed unconscious impulses can be made conscious, psychoanalysis."

"According to Freud, psychoneuroses and many psychoses are

the result of this inability of the patient to face the entirety of his emotional situation. This inability Freud considered as a failure in the highest integrative functions of the personality or, in terms of neurophysiology, of the highest integrating centres of the brain."

Freud's phylogenetic thinking never left him, and it may have been one of the most useful things which he carried with him from his undergraduate medical education. Certainly his early practice in drawing generalizations from his observations stood him well in later life. From petromyzon to psychoanalysis was a long journey, but as Brill concluded, in his excellent biographical study: "Freud had, as it were, started from the ranks, as a private, yet from the beginning he carried the commander's staff in his knapsack."

A prophet without honour in 1886, Freud has nevertheless become a prophet to many, and with reason, as the following extract from his address to the International Psychoanalytic Congress in 1918 suggests:

"But one day the conscience of society will awaken, and we shall realize that . . . man has the same claim to mental treatment that he now has to surgical aid. And we shall also come to see that the neuroses menace the health of the people no less than does tuberculosis, and that, like tuberculosis, the neuroses cannot be left to the ineffectual care of the individual himself. When that time comes, institutes and consultation centres will be established, and staffed with trained physicians, so that men who would otherwise give way to drink, women who would break down as a result of overwhelming deprivations, and children whose choice would be limited to delinquency or neurosis, may be strengthened to resist such unhealthy tendencies and become capable of social achievements."

NEUROPATHOLOGY

The field of neuropathology boasts a trio of student investigators in Schilder, von Monakow and Nissl.

Paul Schilder (1886-1940) made his first contribution in neuropathology while an undergraduate. Two years after graduation he published papers on his research into the anatomical lesions which produce bizarre choreic and athetoid movements. The affliction now called "Schilder's Disease"—encephalitis periaxialis diffusa—he first described in 1912, three years after graduation.

Though extremely well grounded in structural neuropathology he was also a keen student of philosophy and psychology, probably because of his student association with Laurenz Müller, the philosopher, and Exner, the physiologist, in Vienna. From Freud he learned much but he was not a strict adherent to his theories.

Schilder's pen was ever active and his breadth of interest wide. His outstanding contribution, he felt, was his *Das Körperschema*—published in Berlin in 1923, and translated as *The Image and Appearance of the Human Body*, in London, in 1935. He died in 1940, struck down by an automobile in New York City.

The Russian-born Constantin von Monakow (1853-1930), who was to become a leader in the field of neurology, and whose life has been so gracefully chronicled by Colin Russel, was a student who fled from the wax models of neuroanatomy after attending only three lectures, to be caught in the mesmerizing web of neuropathology. As a psychiatric student on Hitzig's wards at Zurich, he was allowed to work over the neurological specimens from the autopsy room. It was in his sixth semester that von Monakow started on histological studies on the brain in dementia.* Interestingly enough he investigated damage to the cerebral blood vessels, the brain cells and liver in experimental chloroform poisoning. Hitzig, who had just discovered the electrical excitability of parts of the cerebral cortex, was so impressed with von Monakow's organizing ability, as a student, that he sent him on a tour of investigation and study of mental institutions. In Munich, von Monakow saw von Gudden's anatomical methods, his microtome, and his set of serial sections of the human brain. This fired his imagination, and took him out of the field of neuropathology and into that of cortical localization of function, his greatest work. His discoveries bear out the thesis that a student can be stimulated to do original research, given the means.

Von Monakow's life illustrates the value to a researcher of

---

* The distinguished Italian neurohistologist, Camillo Golgi (1844-1926), in his graduation thesis at Pavia (1865) wrote a critical review on the need for a classification of mental diseases according to (a) microscopic structural changes in the brain, and (b) causal factors.

sufficient isolation from the busy world to enable him to concentrate on tough problems for long periods at a time. The seven most productive years of von Monakow's life were spent in an old Benedictine monastery which had become a mental hospital, in St. Gaul in Switzerland. For his microscopic studies he sectioned brains which had been hardened in formaldehyde and fixed in chromic acid. These were held firmly in a mixture of pig's fat and suet, within a metal cylinder, while the very thin sections were cut with a two-handled draw-knife under water. It was with such primitive equipment and far away from any cultural centres that this dynamic man demonstrated some of the cardinal truths of modern neurology. We often forget what first class discoveries have been made by physicians isolated in rural mental institutions. In such surroundings A. W. Campbell, the Australian, spent thirteen years as resident medical officer and pathologist in an asylum in the Liverpool area while he produced his great atlas on the microscopic structure of the brain's surface. His maps are used today wherever the brain is studied.*

Franz Nissl (1860-1919), after deserting theology and gaining a medical education after much privation, made his first contribution at the age of 24 in Munich when, in a prize-winning dissertation, he analyzed "The pathological changes of the Nerve Cells of the Cerebral Cortex." Using alcohol-fixed brains and by staining with magenta red (a forerunner of the blue dyes now associated with his name) he showed many new details of the finer structure of nerve cells. Such was his student reputation that he was taken into von Gudden's Institute and given a laboratory and assistants immediately upon graduation.

Every medical student learns early in his career about "Nissl

* Weigert, Ehrlich and Edinger were chiefs of the respective sections of the Senckenbergisches Pathologisch-Anatomisches Institut at Frankfurt-am-Main, which under their guidance became famous. The "Institut" was actually "an ill-equipped old private cottage," but it united the efforts of three productive giants in medical research.

The Nobel laureate Camillo Golgi began his research career while resident physician to a chronic hospital in Abbiategrasso, a small Italian town devoid of scientific or academic contacts. He worked at night in the kitchen of his home, by candlelight. There in 1873 he discovered his silver chromate method for staining the minute structures of the nervous system—a method still producing new and beautiful vistas under the microscope today.

granules"—those "spots on the tiger's skin" which indicate so delicately the state of health of a nerve cell. The reactions to injury of the cell or of its conducting process—the axone—are easily-read barometers which have aided in thousands of researches since Nissl's earliest descriptions. It is a shame that all medical students could not have known Franz Nissl as well as his "granules," for he was a man full of humour, an excellent pianist and a deflater of his overly serious colleagues. The late A. T. Rasmussen used to tell of Nissl's endless teasing of his friend and colleague Kraepelin—the psychiatrist, full of brilliance but also of distractions. Nissl would arrange an armful of beerbottles outside a suitable laboratory, informing all who passed that there was serious inebriety abroad in the department, headed, of course, by the militant crusader against alcoholism, Kraepelin himself.

Nissl had a technique for winnowing down the number of students who sought interviews. Only the truly serious ones ever saw him—for he saw them "at twelve"—meaning midnight, after his patients had been visited, his research concluded for the day, and his favorite sonata played at home in peace. Such was the puckish, human and industrious Franz Nissl. He died at the age of fifty-eight of a chronic kidney ailment.

The contributors to neurology at the clinical level can claim a great many student investigators in their ranks. Osler, Romberg, and Raynaud are discussed elsewhere. Here we shall concentrate on Brissaud, Henri Claude, Babinski, Schaffer, Huntington and Oppenheim. But first let us dwell on a little-known figure, Nathan Strong, Jr., who published a graduation dissertation at Hartford, Connecticut, in 1810, "On the disease termed petechial or spotted fever." It was as important, in its way, as Elisha North's Monograph of 1811 on cerebrospinal meningitis, which is usually quoted as the earliest definitive work.

Edouard Brissaud (1852-1909) lived a life full to overflowing with clinical observations, on paralysis agitans, medico-legal problems in injuries of the nervous system, history, and folklore. His life was cut short by a brain tumor, which was operated upon in Paris by Sir Victor Horsley—alas, too late. As a medical student he began his neurological writings by discussing, as his graduation dissertation, the paralysis which follows a "stroke"—otherwise known as hemiplegia. The permanent contractures which ensued, and which so deformed once-flexible limbs occupied most of his attention. It is interesting, in the light of his later medico-legal writings, that his thesis clearly described a type of periodic or remitting hemiplegia found in lesions of the pons, adjacent to the bulbar area. Brissaud was one of the founders of that bible of French neurology, the *Revue Neurologique.*

The disease multiple sclerosis is well-known today due to strenuous efforts by lay organizations to accelerate research into its cause and possible cure. The youthful Cruveilhier described the structural abnormalities seen in this disease in 1835 in Paris, and it is reported that Robert Carswell as a medical student in London drew colored illustrations of similar spinal cord lesions sometime before 1837. However, these were descriptions only, and not directed towards actual experiments. The first to develop the investigative approach was the medical student Henri Claude (1869-1945), who, working in Bouchard's laboratory in Paris, wrote his thesis on the lesions in the liver, kidneys and nervous system which followed an injection of tetanus and other toxins. The resulting obstruction of the veins in all three tissues has, as Dr. Hyman Morrison writes, "opened up a new approach to the understanding of the etiology of multiple sclerosis." This thesis was so outstanding that it was awarded the Gold Medal of the Hospitals of Paris. For the past sixty years interest has centred on the venous obstruction theory set in motion by Henri Claude.

This neurologist has been inexplicably neglected by historians of medicine. His education was thorough and he came to his chosen work with a brilliant record. On graduation he picked up the threads of his earlier thesis work and pushed ever further into the mysteries of multiple sclerosis, and, of great interest to us in recent years, into the elimination of salt in kidney diseases. He wrote on epilepsy, tumors of the pineal gland—once alleged to be the seat of the soul—tumors of the third ventricle of the brain, the propagation of tumors, and on encephalitis. The first World War brought him into close touch with peripheral nerve injuries and with hysteria.

The measurement of cerebrospinal fluid pressure was of great interest to Claude and he did pioneer work in graphically recording its changes in various postures, after the administration of drugs, and after the compression of the jugular veins. The latter manoeuvre we use daily in searching for spinal cord tumors. He was one of the first to develop an interest in the possible role of the thymus gland in muscle diseases. He also surmised that deep in the hypothalmus—that primitive part of the nervous system just above the pituitary gland—there must be some central representation of the autonomic or involuntary nervous system.

It is little wonder that Claude occupied Charcot's chair in nervous and mental diseases in Paris from 1921 to 1939. He was truly a forerunner of much that is thought to be modern or advanced today. He was a psychobiologist, a good psychiatrist, and a pioneer in preventive mental health services, including the use of psychiatric social workers. His work on experimental epilepsy in animals with brain wounds has a very modern ring to it. Withal he was a very human physician and teacher.

The French interest in multiple sclerosis stems also from J. F. F. Babinski (1857-1932). Every student knows that if a patient's great toe goes up when his foot is stroked he is said to have "Babinski's sign." Few realize that Babinski was once a lowly student too—and that he wrote his graduation thesis for the University of Paris on multiple sclerosis. He had already written a paper on typhoid fever two years previously. At the age of thirty-nine he reported on his "cutaneous plantar reflex," which we now call his sign. This milestone in neurological diagnosis was presented in a communication of only twenty-eight lines. Hundreds of papers and several books have since been written about it by others!

In 1855 Miss Augusta Klumpke (1859-1927) of San Francisco, a student of Dejerine in Paris, first described the paralysis of the arm from a traction injury to the brachial plexus which is still known as "Klumpke's Paralysis." Two years later she became the first woman in France to hold the title "interne des hopitaux" —a matter which raised so much opposition that it was only settled by the Minister of Public Instruction, the physiologist Paul Bert. The following year she married the famous Joseph Jules Dejerine (1849-1917).

The role of heredity and constitution in diseases of the nervous system continues to attract investigators. Two of these, historically, were student contributors. In the case of Karoly Schaffer (1864-1939), the father of Hungarian neurology, the approach to the nervous system was through an undergraduate study which he made of the mechanism involved in the transmission of the virus disease rabies. This early paper was published in Budapest. He carried on post-graduate study in Germany with the versatile Weigert and there encountered Edinger, a brilliant colleague and researcher.

Schaffer's work is reported in two hundred papers which he published. His "triad" of criteria for judging a neurological disease hereditary consisted of (a) a defect in the germ plasm of ectoderm of the developing embryo; (b) localization of symptoms to correspond with the anatomical abnormality; and (c) selectivity of the clinical defect for a specific system or faculty. His last paper was on his hero Semmelweis. He had just put down his pen when the end came, at age seventy-five.

The unique contribution of George Huntington in the field of hereditary diseases of the nervous system we should describe in some detail.

George Huntington (1850-1916)

George Huntington was born in East Hampton, Long Island, New York, on April 9, 1850. His father and grandfather had, in succession, practised medicine in East Hampton for over fifty years. The unique contribution which George Huntington made to medical knowledge is the description of the chorea which we now know by his name. His was not the first description of the disease, but as Osler put it, "In the history of medicine there are few instances in which a disease has been more accurately, or graphically, or more briefly described."

Although it was not until a few months after graduation from the College of Physicians and Surgeons, New York, in 1871, that George Huntington's work appeared in print, he had been a student of chorea since his boyhood. Huntington's own description of how he became interested in the disease and made a study of it throughout his student years, cannot be improved upon. He told the New York Neurological Society on December 7, 1909:

"Over fifty years ago in riding with my father on his professional rounds, I saw my first case of 'that disorder,' which was the way in which the natives always referred to the dreaded disease. I recall it as vividly as though it had occurred but yesterday. It made a most enduring impression upon my boyish mind, an impression every detail of which I recall today, an impression which was the very first impulse to my choosing chorea as my virgin contribution to medical lore. Driving with my father through a wooded road leading from East Hampton to Amagansett, we suddenly came upon two women, mother and daughter, both tall, thin, almost cadaverous, both bowing, twisting, grimacing. I stared in wonderment, almost in fear. What could it mean? My father paused to speak with them, then we passed on. Then my Gamaliel-like instruction began; my medical instruction had its inception. From this point on, my interest in the disease has never wholly ceased."

Huntington's formal description of this type of chorea was read before a Medical Society Meeting on February 15, 1872, in Middleport, Ohio. He had worked on the manuscript while assisting his father at East Hampton, immediately after graduation. Throughout the manuscript are corrections in his father's handwriting. It is little wonder that George Huntington gave such credit to both his grandfather and his father for teaching him what they did, not only about chorea, but about medicine in general. Commenting upon this, George Huntington remarked that, "In old Greece the pupil sat at the feet of his teacher; so your essayist sat at the feet of these two, and whatever of honor, whatever of praise, whatever of scientific worth there is, is due much more to them than to him to whom has come the unsought, unlooked-for honor."

As one reads Huntington's paper today one can hardly believe that it was written by a man of twenty-two years. It bears the stamp of long experience which, of course, Huntington as has already been shown, definitely had with this disease. As Osler remarked, "It is truly a classic and has scarcely been improved upon since it was first set down." The following brief extracts from Huntington's original paper may therefore be of interest.

"The *hereditary* chorea, as I shall call it, is confined to certain and fortunately a *few* families, and has been transmitted to them as an heirloom from generations away back in the dim past. It is spoken of by those in whose veins the seeds of the disease are known to exist, with a kind of horror, and not at all alluded to except through dire necessity, when it is mentioned as '*that disorder*.' It is attended generally by all the symptoms of common chorea, only in an aggravated degree, hardly ever manifesting itself until *adult* or *middle* life, and then coming on gradually but surely, increasing by degrees, and often occupying years in its development, until the hapless sufferer is but a quivering wreck of his former self. . . . There are three marked peculiarities in this disease: 1) Its hereditary nature. 2) A tendency to insanity and suicide. 3) Its manifesting itself as a grave disease only in adult life. . . . In all the families, or nearly all in which the choreic taint exists, the nervous temperament greatly preponderates, and in my grandfather's and father's experience, which conjointly covered a period of seventy-eight years, nervous excitement in a marked degree almost invariably attends upon every disease these people may suffer from, although they may not when in health be over nervous. . . . I have never known a recovery or even an amelioration of symptoms in this form of chorea; when once it begins, it clings to the bitter end. No treatment seems to be of any avail, and indeed nowadays its end is so well known to the sufferer and his friends, that medical advice is seldom sought. It seems at least to be one of the incurables."

In addition to the thoroughness and penetrating nature of Huntington's observations as a boy and young man, one is struck by the fact that he noted in his paper the location of the geographical pockets in which his cases were discovered. The leads which he and others gave in this direction were of the greatest value to Macdonald Critchley when he came to draw together, in skillful fashion, the tangled threads of the story of this hereditary chorea.

George Huntington should be remembered as an observant son and grandson of pioneer physicians in a land so long and so well served by its general practitioners.

Congenital abnormalities of the nervous system are of the greatest interest today when we know something of the effects of diseases such as rubella complicating pregnancy. One of the early students of this field was Hermann Oppenheim (1858-1919) who described *amyotonia congenita*—also called Oppenheim's disease. As we pick up a limp, toneless infant with "rubber legs" today we think back to Oppenheim's original cases of the year 1900. We might go further back to his graduation thesis of 1881 on the metabolism of urea in the body. He had already published three papers on this problem while a student so keen was he in physiological pursuits.

NEUROPHYSIOLOGISTS

Finally, the physiologists of the nervous system encompass one of the most influential groups in medical history. Though most of them worked in laboratory sciences their contributions have changed the whole of clinical medicine. In this section only Purkinje, Brown-Sequard and Sherrington will be studied in detail. The lives of Pavlov, Claude Bernard and Cannon have been described in the chapter on digestion.

Johannes Evangelista Purkinje (1787-1869)

Johannes Purkinje was born in Libochovice, Bohemia, and received his early education there from the Piarist monks. He became a novitiate and for three years taught in the school, but then decided to study philosophy in Prague. Lacking any support from home—his father having died in 1797—Johannes became tutor to the family of Baron Hildprandt. The Baron eventually made it possible for Purkinje to take up the study of medicine, and soon we find him engrossed in pharmacological studies, in which he himself was the experimental subject. The interest which he showed in intoxications by belladonna, camphor and other substances was maintained throughout his life.

Under the influence of the poet Goethe's *Farbenlehre*, Purkinje became attracted to visual problems, and for his graduation thesis at Prague, in 1819, wrote a dissertation on "The subjective features of vision." This essay was expanded six years later to include an account of his experimental work on "after-images" and on differences in the threshold of vision for various colors.

The following year Purkinje began his work on dizziness and on the jerking motion of the eyes, known as nystagmus, following rotation of the body, as in a swivel chair. In this, as in many other fields, Purkinje anticipated by many years the workers still regarded in the West as the pioneers or discoverers.

Purkinje was a friend of Goethe, the poet, Hegel the philosopher, and the brothers von Humbolt in Berlin. Together they persuaded the German Government that their brilliant protégé merited a professorship. Accordingly, Purkinje was installed in the chair of physiology in Breslau, in 1823.* Breslau's German University received the young Czech professor in a very cold fashion, and when he started elementary laboratory exercises and demonstrations for the medical students, his colleagues urged upon the government his early removal. The Ministry of Education replied by building him a first class Physiological Institute.

Purkinje ranks as one of the fathers of histology—the science of tissues. He was the first to develop a microtome for cutting thin sections of tissues for microscopic study. This led to important studies in embryology. He discovered the sweat glands of the skin in 1833, and kept up a running fire of researches, assisted always by his students.

In 1835 his wife, a daughter of Rudolphi, the Berlin anatomist, died of "the pest," along with two children. Thereafter Purkinje worked in a small laboratory in his home—much as Ramón y Cajal did in Madrid after a large Institute was built in his honour. From Purkinje's home came many important theses by students, reporting, for the first time, their master's discoveries. Thus Adolph Wendt in his Latin graduation dissertation at Breslau in 1833, *De epidermide humana,* described in detail the opening of the sweat glands on the surface of the human skin. Purkinje had noted contorted and spiral "threads" in the skin but his pupil showed them to be ducts.

In 1837 Purkinje made his great microscopic survey of the substance of the brain, giving the first accurate account of the billions of nerve cells which make it up, together with their nuclei, their receiving apparatuses "the dendrites," and their transmitting fibres, covered with insulation or "myelin." In the cerebellum he

* His inaugural lecture is remarkable for the broad spectrum of interests which it discloses. Besides visual subjects such as dioptrics, it covers skin sensation, and, most importantly, it contains the first mention of fingerprints as having individual characteristics.

described those "flask-shaped ganglionic bodies," known to this day as "Purkinje cells."

More important, however, were his observations in 1837 on the basic similarity in structure between the cells of plant and animal tissues. He laid the groundwork for that great generalization—"the cell theory"—in 1838 by Schleiden and Schwann. In 1839 Purkinje introduced the term "protoplasm" to facilitate discussion of animal tissues, since the physician-botanist Schleiden had used chiefly botanical terminology.

The all-important fibres of the heart which are specialized for electrical conduction—known as the Purkinje fibres—were first described in the thesis, "De musculari cordi structura" (1839) by Bogislaus Palicki, one of Purkinje's students, who gave his master full credit for their discovery. Another student dissertation, "De structura fibrosa uteri nongravidi," by Wilhelm Kasper in 1840, reported the discovery of what we still call the "Purkinje fibres" of the uterus.

No brief sketch can do justice to this remarkable man. His interests ranged from the microscopic structure of the teeth, to that of the skin, bones, blood vessels and seminal vesicles. He did the early basic work on the ciliary motion by which particles are carried along moist epithelial surfaces within the body. He showed that deaf mutes could receive and appreciate the vibrations of a tuning fork in contact with the skull.

A very significant paper was written by Purkinje, in 1846, on dreams as possible indicators of personality structure. Purkinje had already anticipated Barany on nystagmus, Galton on fingerprints, Schleiden and Schwann on cell structure—why not Freud on dreams?

In 1850, at the age of sixty-three, Purkinje was welcomed home to Prague and was given the Chair of Physiology and a good laboratory in which to work. He became a great national figure, known not only for his discoveries, but also for the translations of Shakespeare, Schiller and Tasso which he made into Czech. He lived until 1869, greatly beloved by his people.

Purkinje was more than a great discoverer in physiology who started as a student contributor. He stands as an important representative of a culture in the cockpit of Europe which has thrown up great minds despite the jackbooted barbarians who have washed in waves over it whether their aims were religious or political. The subjection of the Czechs did not prevent John Wycliffe in England from proclaiming John Huss as a great leader. This nation, prostrated twice in ten years by modern police states, should not be forgotten. Purkinje should remain in the minds of freemen of science as a great pioneer and a powerful beacon.

Charles-Edouard Brown-Séquard (1818-1894)

Poets and playwrights are common enough in the annals of French medicine but the playwright Brown-Séquard, successor in the Chair of Medicine at the Collège de France to the playwright Claude Bernard, was no ordinary Frenchman. In fact he was half American. His father was a Philadelphia sea captain, Charles Edward Brown, who sailed into the island of Mauritius, or the Isle de France, in the Indian Ocean, on his merchant ship. There he married Charlotte Séquard, a vivacious French resident. Their "Paul et Virginie" existence was interrupted by a famine which threatened the island and Captain Brown volunteered to sail a ship to India to collect rice. On the return journey the ship foundered with the loss of all on board.

Charles-Edouard was born then into a fatherless world, and had to make his way by working in a shop, while he wrote his plays and poems. His friends saw in him such promise that they financed his passage to Paris, where, discouraged by the critics, as Claude Bernard had been, he burned his manuscripts and entered medicine. To earn a living he tutored other students in his class, for he was well out in front of them in his studies, especially since his gift for writing eased his way at examination time.

Two years before he graduated Brown-Séquard carried on research on the effect of human gastric juice on the food ingested. He swallowed sponges, which, when saturated, were pulled up by a string and the gastric juice collected and tested. His M.D. thesis, presented in 1846, was a remarkable preview of what his life's work was to be. In his own words he described it thus:

> This work is composed of two distinct parts: the first has for its object the study of reflex movements in batrachians, especially the augmentation of the reflex faculty after section of the cord;

> the second treats of the properties and functions of the columns of the cord and has for its chief aim the demonstration that the transmission of sensation is by way of the gray substance and not by the dorsal (posterior) columns. In this second part the author remarks that pricking the anterior columns of the cord in frogs, eels, pigeons, rabbits and dogs causes only local contractions, an important fact which shows the *inexcitability* of the longitudinal fibres of the anterior columns.

Thus we find in his student thesis the germ of his later generalization that a spinal cord lesion produces a distal sensory loss on the opposite side of the body, and a motor deficit on the side of the lesion—the well-known "Brown-Séquard syndrome."

His American heritage may have taken him to Richmond where he held a chair in the University of Virginia. He oscillated back and forth across the Atlantic, being at one time a professor at Harvard. He finally settled at the Collège de France where his life work was done, on the physiology of the nervous system and on the importance of the adrenal glands to survival of animal life.

Sir Charles Sherrington (1857-1952)

The great explorers in history have had rivers, seas and continents named for them. There is probably no single continent in the neurological world large enough to memorialize adequately the name of Charles Scott Sherrington as the explorer of the nervous system. He was a veritable Columbus. His name is associated with so many of the milestones in this sphere that we can well appreciate the truth of the statement, "Sherrington did for the nervous system what Harvey did for the circulatory system."

Sherrington, though born in Islington, was associated throughout his life with Ipswich and the cities of Britain's eastern seaboard. His father died at an early age and his mother later married an Ipswich physician and scholar, Dr. Caleb Rose. Under his tutelage Charles was to develop, with his three brothers, into an active lad with artistic and literary interests, and with a flair for athletics —playing rugby for St. Thomas's Hospital and rowing for Caius College, Cambridge.

Throughout his life Sherrington was interested in the works of the physician-poet John Keats, as his own style of writing would suggest. With a classical education and an interest in science Sherrington found himself doubly prepared for a world which was rapidly changing in philosophical and scientific concepts. One might be talking with him about some occult theory of consciousness when he would suddenly say, "Of course Cicero really expressed it better than we can." He maintained this ability to call on classical allusions to the end of his ninety-five years.

After a false start in medicine at Edinburgh, Sherrington entered Cambridge and there fell under the spell of the great physiologist Michael Foster. As an undergraduate in Foster's laboratory Sherrington was caught up in one of the most interesting scientific controversies of the last century. The question being debated hotly was the existence of localized areas of the brain, specific for each function carried out by the body. The setting for the most forthright exchange of views in this matter was the Seventh International Medical Congress, held in London in 1881.

At this congress Professor Goltz of Strasbourg demonstrated a dog from whose brain he had made large tissue removals, and in whose performance he said he found no change. Goltz therefore concluded that there was no real localization of function in the brain whatever.

Goltz's own estimate of the dog's performance was at once challenged by Gerald Yeo, a surgeon who was at that time Professor of Physiology at King's College, London. Yeo thought the dog did show a deficit, and, in passing, he waxed caustic on the desirability of asepsis in neurosurgery.

Next on the programme came David Ferrier, the neurologist, demonstrating a monkey in which he and Yeo had made a cortical removal seven months previously. As the monkey dragged his limbs along on the side opposite to the removal, the great Charcot remarked, 'C'est un malade." But this was not all. A second monkey was shown, from which the auditory cortex, as we now know it, had been removed on both sides, ten weeks before. Exploding a percussion cap beside it failed to produce any response, and deafness from the cortical removals seemed proven. As tempers rose over the two views—localization or no localization of function—it was suggested that the animals should be chloroformed forthwith and that a representative committee should report on the state of the brains. Only in England would the committee method have suggested itself! At all events one hemisphere of the brain of Goltz's famous dog found its way to Cambridge with J. N. Langley of the Committee, and it was on this specimen that Sherrington the undergraduate was put to work. His first publication with Langley appeared in 1884, and in 1885 Sherrington, alone, published a further work concerning it. Thus C. S. S. found himself afloat on the sea of neurology, with a full tide running.

For a time Sherrington demonstrated in anatomy at Cambridge under Sir George Humphry who said of him at that time: "He did his work well and the students were much attached to him. His genial friendly qualities made him a general favorite and a most agreeable colleague." Proceeding to St. Thomas' Hospital Medical School, London, where he had had his name on the register for some time, Sherrington carried on with his formal medical course, while demonstrating in histology. He qualified as M.R.C.S. in the latter part of 1884 and proceeded to Strasbourg to work with Goltz at first hand.

Returning to Cambridge he completed his M.B. degree with distinction and began his study of pathology. On a combined Cambridge University-Royal Society study of cholera, he, J. Graham Brown and C. S. Roy were sent to Spain to investigate claims that a vaccine against the disease had been perfected. They made many interesting observations and post-mortem examinations, but found the vaccine non-existent. In later years it was like a chapter out of *Don Quixote* and his windmills to hear Sir Charles relate the comic opera nature of parts of this adventure.

A year later he travelled to Italy to investigate another outbreak, and, of course, used the opportunity very wisely to visit art galleries and libraries also. (It was probably here that he contracted that expensive disease for which there is no cure, bibliophilia. It has since proven highly infectious, especially among neurologists.)

Sherrington took some of his pathological material to Berlin to examine in the laboratory of Rudolf Virchow, another of our student contributors. Virchow's life as a pathologist was almost over, so deeply had he become immersed in German politics.

Although Sherrington found it more profitable to transfer to Robert Koch's laboratory, he nevertheless admired the manner in which Virchow stood up to Bismarck. Strasbourg had opened Sherrington's eyes to the jackboot of Prussianism, and he never forgot it. During the First World War and throughout the Nazi Invasion of Spain beginning in 1936, Sherrington cursed the German dictators.

One apocryphal story is told in which Sherrington, early in 1914, sent some microtome knives to the Sartorious factory in Göttingen for re-sharpening. The war intervened and for four years Sherrington repeated ruefully his certainty that the steel blades had been turned into weapons to kill his countrymen. At the end of the war the resharpened blades were returned by post, with a note: "Due to unforeseen circumstances delivery has been delayed."

Instead of a proposed stay of six weeks in Koch's laboratory Sherrington remained until the following year, learning microscopic anatomy and bacteriology, which were to be of the greatest use to him later. While in Berlin he heard lectures by Helmholtz, DuBois-Reymond, and Waldeyer. He dismissed the latter as superficial when he pointed out a nerve cell to Sir Charles as "Das Denkorgan." Waldeyer's later popularization of already known facts as the "Neurone Theory" annoyed Sherrington mightily, and he always came vehemently to the defence of Cajal and Van Gehuchten as the real authors of the theory.

Returning to England, Sherrington was made a lecturer in physiology at St. Thomas' Hospital Medical School. At the end of the year he was named Professor-Superintendent of the Brown Institution of the University of London as successor to Sir Victor Horsley. (This remarkable veterinary laboratory for the care of sick animals and for research into their diseases, was established by the will of Thomas Brown in 1852, but nineteen years of discussion ensued before it was constructed.) In this setting Sherrington was to carry out some of his greatest detective work on the secrets of the nervous system. In probing the knee-jerk, he sought answers to the question: How did the spinal cord cause certain muscles to contract, extending the knee, when the patellar tendon was tapped? He discovered that nerves connecting muscles to the spinal cord were approximately one-third sensory in function, and only two-thirds motor (i.e., causing contractions). Why were there sensitive fibres carrying messages *from* muscles *to* the nervous system? This Sherrington answered with a series of remarkable papers on the microscopic pressure and tension receptors concealed within limb muscles. Thereafter, an explanation of posture became possible.

Sherrington ushered in the use of diphtheria antitoxin in Britain in a remarkable incident. He had been immunizing a horse when news reached him that his nephew on the south coast had contracted the disease. He bled the horse and rushed serum to the patient in time to save his life. Lister was greatly excited by all this, told to him the same evening.

The University of Liverpool appointed Sherrington to the Holt Chair of Physiology in 1895, and in that capacity he was to become one of the outstanding writers on science in the English-speaking world. With Harvey Cushing he explored electrically the surface of the brain in orang-utangs, gorillas and chimpanzees. His discoveries required the coining of new terms which would be exact and not confusable. The early training at Ipswich Grammar School in language was to guide Sherrington in his choice of such terms as "synapse," "decerebrate rigidity" and "the final common pathway." His Silliman Lectures given at Yale University in 1904 advanced our knowledge still further as he described "The Integrative Action of the Nervous System."

The Liverpool period was rich in discoveries made and life-long friendships developed, such as that with the pioneer American neurosurgeon Harvey Cushing. Sherrington's boyish appearance and cycling were probably surprises to Cushing, who was fascinated by the gold spectacles perched precariously on the physiologist's nose, even when he had "lost" them.

The working out of the segmental arrangements within the nervous system, of the reciprocal action of antagonistic muscles, and reflex inhibition, all occurred in this fruitful period. Sherrington astounded some physiologists when he wrote that "Desistence from action may be as truly active as is the taking of action." He welded together neurophysiology and neuroanatomy at every turn, and in no place more successfully than at the "synapse" (from the Greek "clasp"), whose activity, multiplied by hundreds of times, gave rise to the "central excitatory state" or to the "central inhibitory state."

Sherrington often returned to his undergraduate work from Cambridge days, concerning the great centrifugal motor pathway, from the brain's surface to the cells of the spinal cord, known as the "pyramidal tract." So in succession came the experiments on "tonus," "decerebrate rigidity" and "the stretch reflex" which are known today, wherever neurology is practised, as the cornerstones.

In 1913 Sir William Osler, Regius Professor of Medicine at Oxford, convinced the board of electors that they should bring Sherrington to fill the Waynflete Professorship of Physiology there. The bibliophiles in Oxford, the humanists, the philosophers and most of all the students applauded this wise decision, for no single appointment did more to change Cecil Rhodes' gloomy prediction that there would never be an Oxford man at the top of the scientific tree. In the years 1913 to 1935 Sherrington had a succession of pupils who went to the top of the tree in many parts of the world: Penfield from America, Cairns, Eccles and Florey from Australia, Denny-Brown from New Zealand, Granit from Finland and John Fulton from the United States, to name but a few.

When World War I broke upon the world C.S.S. went on a mission for the War Office—to work as an unskilled laborer in a munitions factory, investigating fatigue. No one in the factory knew him, and when he left after three months, the foreman offered him a letter of reference should he ever need it! His report that a 13-hour day, which he (aged 57) and his unskilled colleagues had worked, was too long to be efficient, eventually found a sympathetic acceptance.

The end of the War brought Sherrington a well-earned period of "diastole" after four years of concentrated "systole," and he was able to write his revolutionary book *Mammalian Physiology: A course of practical exercises.* A foreign reviewer complained that the examples in the book were taken from English authorities only—little realizing that the data were those collected by physiology students in the laboratory at Oxford over the previous seven years.

The years between the wars were to be Sherrington's happiest and busiest. From 1920 to 1925 he served as President of the Royal Society, and found time to publish his remarkable "Assaying of Brabantius and other verse." Some few have heard of it, but fewer still had a chance to savour its contents. Two short selections may give the reader pleasure:

NOW IN THE CLOISTER FEW THE FEET THAT ROAM

Now in the cloister few the feet that roam,
ours that must stay, who little can than wait,
exchange our tidings, good, ill, early, late,
and send our 'god-speed' to them past the foam,
the young folk, splashed with death in the trenched
loam.
Ay, oil the hinges of the ancient gate,
keep burnished bright the goblet's silvern state
against the hour shall hail the soldier home.
You stately tower, from high you saw them go,
and have full many doughty scenes and fair
watched and swung bells above, shattering the air
to honour heroes, you too wait as though
of our poor hearth-bound presence scarcely ware,
you heard from far the filial bugles blow.

1916

One can imagine Sherrington writing from his College, Magdalen, at the river's edge:

OXFORD

The night is fallen and still thou speakst to me,
what though with one voice sole, with accents many,
tongued turret and tongued stream, tracked pasture fenny,
and cloister spirit trod, and centuried tree,
and, bondsmen loosed in Time's tranquillity,
thy bell-dischargèd hours. If wharfage any
thine 'tis where Age shall, nursing late his penny,
smile at long last to hand him Charon's fee.
And now, below, through shadows starr'd, a boat

steals by me laden with singing and young laughter,
and, higher, a wide-flung casement casts afloat
pulses of waltz the which white robes sway after;
vowed Priest of Beauty, these they shrines among,
thou kneelst with old folk, thou that dancest with young.

Sherrington's literary life ranged from poetry to philosophy. His pupil E. G. T. Liddell relates that a few weeks after the publication of Robert Bridges' *The Testament of Beauty* in 1930, Sherrington, long an admirer of his medical student contemporary, fell to reciting long passages from it while preparing the experimental laboratory for the day's teaching. In the academic term 1937-38, Sherrington gave the Gifford Lectures at Edinburgh, published as *Man on His Nature.* Again because, as literature, this is so narrowly known, let us contemplate an extract from it concerning "the brain and its work":

A scheme of lines and nodal points, gathered together at one end into a great ravelled knot, the brain, and at the other trailing off to a sort of stalk, the spinal cord. Imagine activity in this shown by little points of light. Of these some stationary flash rhythmically, faster or slower. Others are travelling points, streaming in serial trains at various speeds. The rhythmic stationary lights lie at the nodes. The nodes are both goals whither converge, and junctions whence diverge, the lines of travelling lights. The lines and nodes where the lights are, do not remain, taken together, the same even a single moment. There are at any time nodes and lines where lights are not.

Suppose we choose the hour of deep sleep. Then only in some sparse and out of the way places are nodes flashing and trains of light-points running. Such places indicate local activity still in progress. At one such place we can watch the behaviour of a group of lights perhaps a myriad strong. They are pursuing a mystic and recurrent manoeuvre as if of some incantational dance. They are superintending the beating of the heart and the state of the arteries so that while we sleep the circulation of the blood is what it should be. The great knotted headpiece of the whole sleeping system lies for the most part dark, and quite especially so the roof-brain. Occasionally at places in it lighted points flash or move but soon subside. Such lighted points and moving trains of lights are mainly far in the outskirts, and wink slowly and travel slowly. At intervals even a gush of sparks wells up and sends a train down the spinal cord only to fail to arouse it. Where however the stalk joins the headpiece, there goes forward in a limited field a remarkable display. A dense constellation of some thousands of nodal points bursts out every few seconds into a short phase of rhythmical flashing. At first a few lights, then more, increasing in rate and number with a deliberate crescendo to a climax, then to decline and die away. After due pause the efflorescence is repeated. With each such rhythmic outburst goes a discharge of trains of travelling lights along the stalk and out of it altogether into a number of nerve-branches. What is this doing? It manages the taking of our breath the while we sleep.

Should we continue to watch the scheme we should observe after a time an impressive change which suddenly accrues. In the great head-end which has been mostly darkness spring up myriads of twinkling stationary lights and myriads of trains of moving lights of many different directions. It is as though activity from one of those local places which continued restless in the darkened main-mass suddenly spread far and wide and invaded all. The great topmost sheet of the mass, that where hardly a light had twinkled or moved, becomes now a sparkling field of rhythmic flashing points with trains of travelling sparks hurrying hither and thither. The brain is waking and with it the mind is returning. It is as if the Milky Way entered upon some cosmic dance. Swiftly the head-mass becomes an enchanted loom where millions of flashing shuttles weave a dissolving pattern, always a meaningful pattern though never an abiding one; a shifting harmony of sub-patterns. Now as the waking body rouses, sub-patterns of this great harmony of activity stretch down into the unlit tracks of the stalk-piece of the scheme. Strings of flashing and travelling sparks engage the lengths of it. This means that the body is up and rises to meet its waking day.

Dissolving pattern after dissolving pattern will, the long day through, without remission melt into and succeed each other in this scheme by which for the moment we figure the brain and spinal cord. Especially, and with complexity incredible, in that part which we were thinking of, the roof-brain. Only after day is done will it quiet down, lapse half-way to extinction, and fall again asleep. Then at last, so far at least as the roof-brain, motor acts cease. The brain is released from the waking day and marshals its factors for its motor acts no more.

Some thought these lectures his "testament of age." Not so those who read them; nor were they surprised to learn of a revised edition being issued in 1951 when C.S.S. was ninety-four. The central figure of the early lectures, Jean Fernel (1497-1557), the first physiologist and pathologist, was further studied in Sherrington's delightful *Endeavour of Jean Fernel* published in 1946 (p. 236).

At the age of ninety-two Sir Charles spoke over the B.B.C. in a symposium on "The physical basis of mind," and listeners will not soon forget the chuckle in his voice as he referred chidingly to some penny-in-the-slot theories of thought processes!

Honours failed to change the charming simplicity of this great man. He was awarded the Order of Merit in 1924, and it would have delighted him to know that after his death his place in this illustrious order, limited to a handful of scholars, was to be taken by his pupil Wilder Penfield.

Today the wheel has come full circle and the study which Sherrington made as an undergraduate in 1885 is the basis of today's neurosurgical operation of "hemispherectomy" to relieve certain cases of cerebral palsy.

Thus, does our generation profit by the work of this gifted medical student born a hundred years ago. As Sir Russell Brain's tribute, read at the Royal College of Physicians, expressed it:

> Yet he was the most modest of men who felt, like Newton, that he had done no more than pick up a few pebbles on the shore of the great ocean of truth.

PLATE 8

(a) Sir Charles Sherrington, O.M. From the portrait by R. G. Eves. Courtesy of The Royal Society, London.

(b) Johannes Evangelista Purkinje (1787-1869). From: Haymaker, Webb: *The Founders of Neurology*, 1953. Courtesy of Charles C Thomas, Publisher.

(c) Sigmund Freud (1856-1939). From: Garrison, Fielding: *History of Medicine*, 1921. Courtesy of W. B. Saunders Co., Publisher.

(d) George Huntington at the age of twenty-two. Courtesy of Prof. Russell De Jong, University of Michigan.

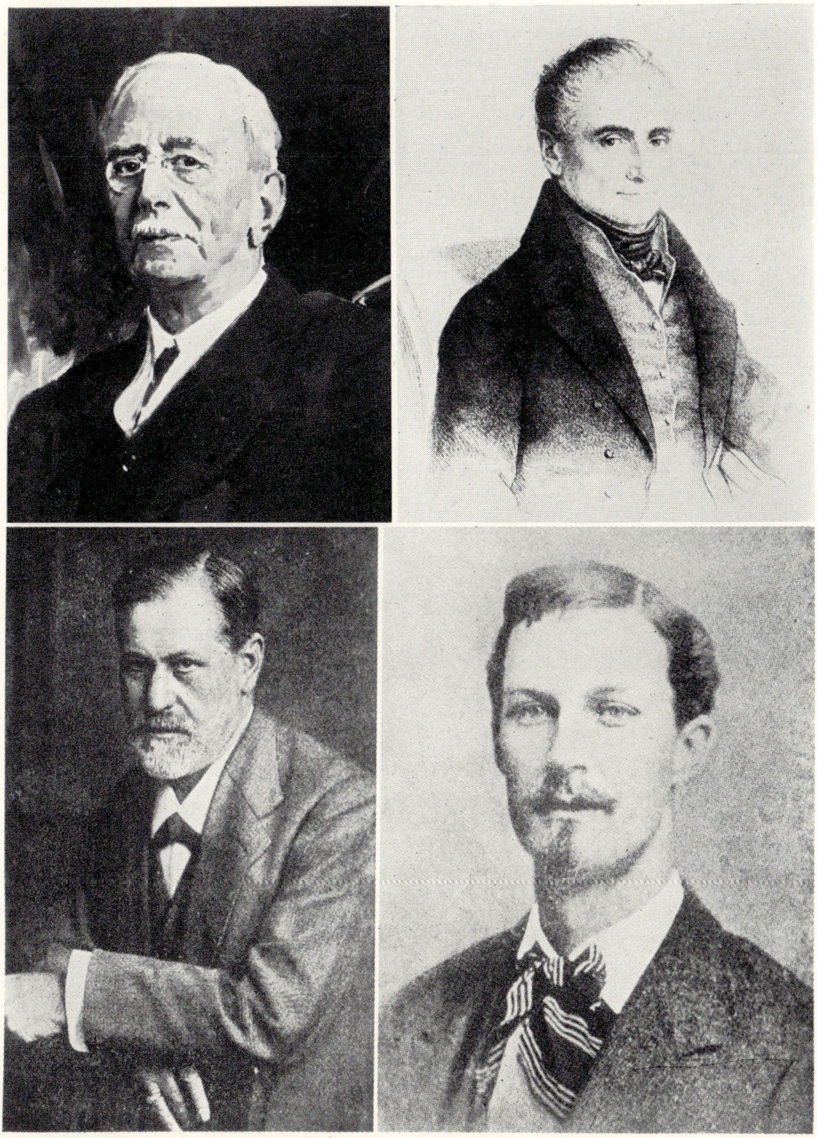

←

Chapter XI

Physics and Optics

Jean Fernel (1497-1557)

JEAN FERNEL was born in 1497 in Montdidier in the diocese of Amiens. His father was a substantial innkeeper and a furrier as well. When Jean was twelve years of age his family moved to Clermont in Beauvoisis, a distance of twenty miles from Paris. After a thorough schooling there, he proceeded, with his father's help, to the University of Paris, entering the progressive Collège de Ste. Barbe, the history of which dated from 1460, when it was established by the Collège de Navarre.

Fernel took his master's degree in Arts, at the age of twenty-two. He was invited to join the faculty of the College and teach Dialectics but he declined. The recent advent of printing had brought the great books within reach of many for the first time and Fernel chose, rather, to learn more of the humanities. The further he went with his self-education the more violently he reacted to his recently "completed" training. He classed some of his tutors as "barbaric," and resolved to go back over all his work systematically and alone. For five years he did nothing but devour "humane letters" and treatises on mathematics. He drove himself so hard that he was taken ill with a "quartan fever," and required a long convalescence.

At the age of twenty-seven he embarked upon the four-year course in medicine at the University of Paris. He had serious financial difficulties since his father could no longer support him, there being others in the family in need of education. As a result, Fernel gave lectures in philosophy at the Collège de Ste. Barbe in order to support himself. As a third year medical student he published his first book, "Monalosphaerium," in which he described an astrolabe which he had invented for calculating the hour of the day, and for measuring elapsed time. This work contains a considerable amount of what we could term astrology today, but which in 1527 was thought to represent the necessary setting for such discussions. Fernel composed an album of illustrations to accompany the main volume.

In the final year of the medical course, Fernel produced his second book entitled *Cosmotheoria.* It is chiefly remembered by mathematicians for the measurement of a degree of meridian which Fernel made from his own observations and his triangulation covering the territory lying between Paris and Amiens. One hundred forty years later Jean Picard was to establish a value almost identical through observations made in the same part of the countryside.

In the same year (1528) Fernel's third book appeared, *De Proportionibus*, in which he discourses on the theory and use of fractions.

In 1530 he received his license to practice. His biographer records: "Fernel's practice became very large. It left him scant time even for his mid-day meal. His patients were of diverse rank, attendants of the court, dignitaries, officials and visitors to Paris, and many of the poor. He never neglected the poor."

Fernel wrote many medical books, among them an *Anatomy*, of which Sherrington says, "The absence of 'pictures' from Fernel's 'Anatomy' may be connected with Fernel's expressed opinion, reported by Plancy, that young physicians mis-spend hours in looking at pictures in anatomy books when, what should be done was to go to actual dissections with a concise manual in the hand. Fernel made his 'Anatomy' a concise manual. It was a preface to his account of the working of the body. Anatomy is to physiology, he says, as geography is to history, it describes the theatre of events."

His textbook on *Physiology*—to use the term which he coined—was a most popular book, and even posthumously thirty-one editions of it were issued over a one-hundred year period. Embarking on something akin to a modern system of medicine, he produced his *Pathology* and *Therapeutics*. His special pathology would strike us today as being very modern. Even in the eighteenth century Boerhaave was still recommending Fernel's pathology as the best available. Thirty-six editions of it were to appear over the next century.

At his death, Fernel left a manuscript on Syphilis, which did not reach a printer's hand until 1579 unfortunately. He complained that the French called it the Neopolitan disease and the Neopolitans called it the French disease. Because printing was becoming widespread, many of the victims of the disease wrote poems on their symptoms and miseries, dedicating them to cardinals and rulers—which led among other things to the erroneous view that it was a disease of poets. Fernel put an end to this sort of pseudo-scientific speculation in his work *De Luis Venereae Curatione*.

Fernel's life in medicine is one of the most absorbing in the history of science, and has been brought before us in the delightful volume by Sir Charles Sherrington, O.M., published in 1946. The restless spirit and the drive to probe into causes, which so possessed Fernel as a student, persisted throughout his life. His simply-stated views have a modern ring to them.

Fernel was not a fractious medical reformer nor political gadfly. He was an excellent and busy practising physician who was indefatigable in his teaching of students. A description of Fernel's day, by his biographer Plancy, reads: "Four o'clock found him risen and in his study, to read or write until daybreak. Then he went out, to visit patients or to the School to lecture. Then back to his study until the midday meal, which he sometimes did not sit down to take. The meal over, he was off again, to visit the sick. At the day's end he supped with his family and after that withdrew again to his study to read or write. He went to bed at one hour before midnight."

In concluding these notes on Fernel's life it might be well to quote some of his pithy remarks. "Many tell us that the art of healing, discovered by the labours of our forefathers, and brought to completion by dint of Reason, has now attained its goal. They would have us, who command it, tread in the same footsteps as did the Past. It were a crime, they tell us, to swerve a hair's breadth from the well established way. But what if our elders, and those who preceded them, had followed simply the same path as did those before them? . . . Nay, on the contrary, it seems good for philosophers to move to fresh ways and systems; good for them to allow neither the voice of the detractor, nor the ways of ancient culture, nor the fullness of authority to deter those who would declare their own views. In that way each age produces its own crop of new authors and new arts. . . . This age need not in any respect despise itself and sigh for the knowledge of the ancients. The orator of today attains the height of oratory. Philosophy excels in every branch. Once again music, geometry, the handicrafts, painting, architecture, sculpture, and many other kinds of skills display themselves in such measure as in no wise to fall short of the achievements of antiquity, which won universal praise. . . . Our age today is doing things of which antiquity did not dream. Antiquity held Demetrius high for engines of war, but today we have petards which hurl a flaming bomb. Good God, how destructive and swift compared with the old catapult! How efficient today the printing-press for the diffusion of all kinds of learning. Today we have paper, once called Fabriano, supplanting wax, bark and skin. Hence, 'letters' today reach their highwater mark. Ocean has been crossed by the prowess of our navigators, and new islands found. The far recesses in India lie revealed. The continent of the West, the so-called New World, unknown to our forefathers, has in great part become known. In all this, and in what pertains to astronomy, Plato, Aristotle and the old philosophers made progress and Ptolemy added a great deal more. Yet, were one of them to return today, he would find geography changed past recognition. A new globe has been given us by the navigators of our time."

Concerning medicine as a calling, Fernel wrote, "Is there a greater blessing vouchsafed to mankind than Medicine is? Life is our dearest possession, by which we breathe and enjoy the company of our fellow-beings. Can any calling be worthier than that which preserves and maintains life itself? Is wealth or fortune, in whatever measure, in the last resort more estimable than is good health? Is any misfortune or disaster more grievous than ill-health? He who succours the sufferer and the sick exercises a knowledge which deserves the admiration and affectionate regard of all men."

Concerning eugenics he wrote: "These beginnings of our being are therefore of much matter to us. Those of us who are endowed with health in virtue of our birth are not a little fortunate. It would be a great good for our race if solely those who are sane and sound gave themselves to the making of children. The husbandman knows that in sowing the land the best seed is to be chosen. Experience has taught him that from poor seed he can expect only a miserly harvest. How much more strictly should that precept be practised in the propagations of our species?"

We can only conclude with Sir Charles Sherrington: "He was one of the relatively few who as they enter advanced years grow more modern."

Galileo Galilei (1564-1642)

Galileo was born 15 February 1564, at Pisa, the eldest of seven children. Many of his ancestors had been physicians. His father was a musician, mathematician and linguist. His early education was at Pisa and at the age of twelve he was sent to school at Vallombrosa near Florence for study in the humanities. Thus was laid a good basis in Greek and Latin and in the natural sciences and philosophy. Galileo became a novitiate of the order which maintained the school at Vallombrosa but his father withdrew him and sought to raise him for the cloth trade of Florence. However, the precocious boy was already well known as a maker of toy machines and models of great ingenuity. He had also learned to play the organ and the lute. He had developed certain skill in drawing and painting and in later life seems to have been a most helpful critic to rising painters. He wrote poetry, essays on Dante and Tasso as well as a play.

The father next looked to a scientific career for his son and because he thought medicine offered some financial stability, he enrolled him in the medical school of the University of Pisa on

September 5, 1581, at the age of seventeen years. The father tried unsuccessfully to get one of the forty free places for needy students at the University in Galileo's first year and again in the third year. Galileo's first contact at the medical school was with the great physician-botanist Andrea Cesalpino, who taught as Professor of Medicine at Pisa from 1567-1592.

Galileo was certainly a discerning student and sought proof of everything. In this he reflected his father's temperament for the father had already stated in some works of literary criticism, "It appears to me that they who, in proof of any assertion, rely simply on the weight of authority, without adducing any argument in support of it, act very absurdly. I, on the contrary, wish to be allowed freely to question and freely to answer, without any sort of adulation, as well becomes those who are sincerely in search of truth."

It is little wonder that his fellow students called Galileo "The Wrangler." He applied his own yardstick to Aristotle, Plato and St. Thomas Aquinas—not a popular pastime with those in authority. As one biographer said, "A philosopher needed only to *know* Aristotle by heart; to *understand* him was a secondary consideration; to *contradict* him was blasphemy."

Galileo made his earliest scientific discovery as a first year medical student in 1581. In the great cathedral of Pisa he saw the lamplighter pull back a large hanging lamp in order to light it. Once lit it was allowed to swing freely in the air. Galileo noticed that though the pendular excursions diminished gradually, the duration of each excursion remained the same. He proved this by reference to his pulse, his only time piece. He experimented at the home of Muzio Tedaldi, a relative with whom he lived in Pisa. There Galileo devised his Pulsilogia, also known as the Protoclock. This had an immediately favorable reception from the physicians of Pisa.

Drawings of three models of Galileo's Pulsilogia are shown below in Plate 9 and were taken from the work of Sanctorius, the founder of the physiology of metabolism and Professor of Medicine at Padua, who in 1607 incorporated them in his book, *Methodi Vitandorum Errorum in Arte Medica.* Fahie's description may be quoted: "Figure 1 consists merely of a weight at the end of a string, which is held at the top of a graduated scale. The string being gathered up into the hand until the vibrations of the weight coincide with the beatings of the patient's pulse, the length is ascertained from the scale, which if great indicates a languid, and if small a more lively action. In figure 2, the improvement is introduced of connecting the scale and string; the length of the latter is regulated by turning a peg, and a bead on the string shows the measure. Figure 3 is still more compact, the string being adjusted by winding or unwinding upon an axle at the back of the dial plate."

In the year 1582-83 Galileo listened to lectures at Pisa by a Florentine friend of his father's, Ostilio Ricci, a mathematician and tutor to the Court of Tuscany. Soon Euclid replaced Hippocrates and Galen in Galileo's interests. Galileo's father set out to prevent any further shift towards mathematics by his son. He petitioned the Grand Duke Fernando I a second time for help for his son from the foundation for poor scholars but to no avail. This may have been due by then to the unpopularity of "The Wrangler" with officialdom. Thus by the summer of 1585 Galileo was withdrawn from the University of Pisa without his degree and he returned home to Florence. There he plunged into mathematics and physics and examined in great detail the works of Archimedes.

In 1586 he constructed his hydrostatic balance with which to analyze alloys. This is reminiscent of Archimedes' detection of fraud by the goldsmith who was making Hiero's crown long since. Galileo then turned to his work on the centre of gravity in solid bodies. His paper brought him immediate and favorable notice in Italy. Despite this the next two years were to see five unsuccessful applications made by him for Chairs of Physics which were vacant. As a result Galileo made ready to set out with another Florentine for the East, when he was accepted at the University of Pisa as a professor with the annual salary of £13.0.0!

Once installed at Pisa, Galileo began to re-examine the teachings of Aristotle in science. Leonardo da Vinci had, unknown to Galileo, done just this. Aristotle's teaching, which was nearly two thousand years prior to Galileo, was that if a heavier and a lighter piece of the same material were dropped from a height simultaneously, the heavier piece would strike the ground first.

Galileo went up to the top of the leaning Tower of Pisa one morning, while students and professors crowded around. He rolled a ten pound shot and a one pound shot over the overhanging edge simultaneously. They struck the ground together, disproving Aristotle's view.

There was, in this demonstration, no timing problem. However, when Galileo sought to prove experimentally that in falling the final velocities are proportional to the times, and the spaces fallen through are proportional to the squares of the times, he had to find an accurate way of measuring time, and for this he went back to his student invention, the Pulsilogia.

Before Galileo's analysis of Aristotle's theories had proceeded much further the spastic minds of Pisa proceeded to castigate Galileo. Galileo went on to ever greater triumphs at Padua, and Pisa forgot their brilliant young scholar. As late as 1613 Father Castelli, Galileo's first pupil, wrote to him from Pisa, "Of our controversies (on the earth's motion) not a word is allowed to be said, a thing which astonishes me. Your marvellous discoveries are scarcely known here even by name."

Galileo's later works on the telescope, the microscope, the thermometer, geometrical and military compasses, fortifications, mechanics and especially astronomy are not within the scope of such a volume as the present but are the basis of his fame as a great contributor to science. Suffice it to say that his observations on natural phenomena and their forthright interpretations brought him into conflict with all manner of entrenched temporal power. Some who had their tenuous theories rocked to the foundations by Galileo's discoveries, accused him of "blasphemy." Others, perceiving the great worth of his inventions and generalizations, stole them! Much of his time was spent in self-defence and in proving plagiarism by his academic colleagues!

The University Senate in Padua, under great pressure in 1599, gave Galileo a niggardly increase in his stipend, from 300 to 320 ducats annually, observing that, "the professors should eke out their income by their private lessons." In addition they told Galileo that, "The Senate does not choose to make his case a precedent for every learned and needy foreigner who might think fit to press his claims, and that the usage of Bologna with regard to her professors was not to be set up as an example, as Bologna had a larger amount of money at the disposal of her University than the Venetian capital Senate had." This has almost a modern ring.

Galileo was twice called before the Inquisition for his Copernican views on the earth's status in the universe and was imprisoned at the age of sixty-eight. All his works were proscribed. This, too, has a modern ring. Borelli, of whom we shall hear again, considered himself a pupil or disciple of Galileo, although he had never seen him. He came from Messina to visit him just before he died. Galileo died on January 8, 1642, surrounded by his son Vincenzio and his wife, by Toricelli, his long and faithful disciple, and the youthful Viviani who was to be his first biographer. Even in death Galileo was further persecuted and his friends were forbidden to bury him in consecrated ground. In 1683 Viviani dared to erect the first memorial to Galileo, and when Viviani died in 1703 he left all his estate for the building of a further memorial. Thirty years more were to elapse before it was thought safe to proceed with this.

Such was the life of Galileo, medical student, astronomer, and physicist who was to pave the way for such scholars as Isaac Newton.

Thomas Young (1773-1829)

In every age there is a rare individual who stands out as a universal genius, gifted in many directions, and able to penetrate with clarity and apparent simplicity the very depths of little-understood secrets of Nature. Thomas Young was such a giant and his Cambridge student title, "Phenomenon Young," fits him well. He enters our field of interest because of a discovery made in his first year in medical school. In 1793 he began his studies in the Great Windmill Street school of John Hunter in London—the last year of Hunter's unparalleled life. By September of 1793 Young had moved over to St. Bartholomew's Hospital Medical School and was dissecting the freshly removed eye of an ox when he observed that the ciliary muscles (later to be described microscopically by another student, Joseph Lister) were still active and, on being stimulated to contract, changed the shape of the lens. This acute observation by an alert and receptive undergraduate brought to an end the spurious though official view, taught for centuries, that focussing of vision on near and distant objects was achieved by a shortening and lengthening of the eyeball itself. The publication of this remarkable discovery earned him his Fellowship in the Royal Society of London at the age of twenty-one.

After a year in London Young decided to enter the Medical School in Edinburgh and there began his studies under Joseph Black the chemist—that quiet, simple man who lived only to discover and to train discoverers, as we have seen in a previous chapter. On his journey to the north Young visited Erasmus Darwin and stopped in Leicestershire to learn the newest methods of stall-feeding cattle, of cross-breeding sheep for wool or for meat, and of irrigating the land. These pursuits by a medical student may strike us as unusual but Young was no ordinary mortal. His pre-medical studies had not been dictated by a few terse lines in a hurdle-listing catalogue of some stone-faced university. As a small boy he had been introduced to oriental studies, Hebrew, colour-mixing, book-binding and copper-plate making. Later his summers were spent with his grandfather in measuring the height of hills with a quadrant, in lens grinding, lathe turning, in making his own microscope and in meteorological observations. Before going up to London from his native Somersetshire he studied French, Persian, Chaldee, Syriac and Samaritan for good measure, together with botany, chemistry, optics and mathematics! With all these accomplishments it is little wonder that Young was sought by the Duke of Richmond, Master-General of Ordnance, as his private secretary, a post which would have foreshortened his career, as such posts seem always to do.

In Edinburgh Young's medical studies were spiced with considerable literary activity. He had already turned his hand to translating Shakespeare into Greek, and now he assisted the Professor of Classics in editing an *Anthology of Greek Poets.*

Before long Young decided that a doctoral degree in medicine from a German university had much to recommend it and he therefore enrolled at Göttingen for his clinical work. He has recorded an example of one of his student days there, which included: History of Europe, materia medica, acute diseases, dancing lessons, music lessons on the clavichord, drawing, physics and medicine. This busy round did not keep him from original work, however, and his thesis, on the human voice, was a remarkable study of sounds of all sorts. The culmination of his experimental work was his presentation of a universal alphabet, comprising forty-seven letters. The combinations of these letters would, he held, reproduce any sound which the human voice could utter. The importance of this invention lies not in the fact that it predates George Bernard Shaw's alphabet, but rather in the train of thought which it started in Young's ever-fertile mind. He reasoned that the combining of sounds might have a counterpart in the field of light, and this analogy he pursued for much of his remaining life. The laws governing the interference of light, and his theory of colour vision (now referred to as the Young-Helmholtz theory) were to be his greatest contributions to science, and rank with Newton's discoveries.

The presentation of Young's thesis in the public auditorium in Göttingen, together with his oral examinations, led to his degree as "Doctor of Physic, Surgery and Man-midwifery." The oral examination he described thus:

> I made no preparatory study, as is usual here, and also at Edinburgh not uncommon, under the name of grinding. The examination lasted between four and five hours; the four examiners were seated round a table, well furnished with cakes, sweetmeats and wine, which helped to pass the time agreeably; the questions were well calculated to sound the depth of a student's knowledge. . . . We were all previously obliged to give a summary account of the manner in which our lives had been spent.

It is remarkable how often Young returned to the question of language and its potentialities in communicating ideas. His apprenticeship as a schoolboy was rich in foreign languages and his work on sound formation and conduction, while a medical student, complemented this early interest. Young did not miss a chance to remark that: "It is also one of the spurious arts of becoming popular, to affect innovations in language," and he said of Emmanuel Kant, "His language is unpardonably obscure." Perhaps Young foresaw the verbal nightmare into which the language of some sciences would degenerate in less salubrious times.

Whatever Young thought of these products of the human

tongue divorced from the brain, he grasped firmly his theory of a universal alphabet tuned to the human ear and representing all possible human voice sounds, usable by all lands. It was therefore no accident that the basalt slab known as the Rosetta Stone, brought to the British Museum after the collapse of Napoleon's forces in Egypt, engaged Young's attention in 1814. It was known that the hieroglyphic inscription was written in 195 B.C., contained a decree by Ptolemy Epiphanes, and had a weathered Greek translation beside it which he was able to handle with ease when it was restored.

Possibly because the hieroglyphs on the stone brought to mind Young's own 47-character alphabet, he made the great initial discovery that Egyptian hieroglyphs were phonetic symbols, and that they were a type of "shorthand for sound." He hastened to apply this to deciphering the Rosetta Stone, and independently discovered the special designations used for proper names and for the name of a goddess. Champollion, usually given credit for these discoveries, actually did his work seven years later.

Prior to this work, however, Young had lived his most productive years. He intended to qualify to practise medicine but the Royal College of Physicians required him to stay two years consecutively in one place! His uncle, Dr. Brocklesby, died leaving him his house in London and £10,000. Young decided to keep his terms at Emmanuel College, Cambridge, returning to London at the end of 1799 to practise in Welbeck Street. It is unlikely that Young spent his time at Cambridge, as it is alleged young men do at Oxford, in "learning to talk nonsense with distinction," for he was soon writing in the Transactions of the Royal Society on his wave theory of light. In his first year of medical practice he wrote the first account of astigmatism.

Young became interested in capillary attraction and from this subject developed his methods of measuring the size of ultimate particles, which as Lord Rayleigh said nearly one hundred years later, clearly establishes Young as the first to measure the size of atoms. He wrote on the theory of the tides, on bridges and construction, giving us Young's modulus which is used daily by engineers in computing the strength and elasticity of materials. He measured the size of the blood corpuscles and of pus cells, and wrote on the dynamics of the blood circulation and the pulse. In the field of life insurance he worked out "A formula for expressing Decrement of Human Life." He standardized the imperial gallon, and contributed to the techniques of gas lighting and of ship-building. He was Secretary of the Board of Longitude, Conductor of the Nautical Almanac, Foreign Secretary of the Royal Society for twenty-seven years and Volta's successor in the French Academy of Sciences.

At the age of thirty-one Young married Eliza Maxwell of Lanarkshire, "a woman of sound common sense." As Sir Thomas Lawrence's portrait, painted three years before Young's death, suggests, he was a handsome man. He was a universal genius, at home in so many fields that we grow breathless in his pursuit. This remarkable man had a great sense of humor as revealed in his letters to friends at home and abroad. No mere summary will do his life justice, but it would doubtless tickle his fancy to know that a sober medical historian of the early part of the twentieth century had concluded that "Young was fond of dancing and good society, but was not regarded as a successful practitioner because he studied symptoms too closely."

Franz Cornelius Donders (1818-1889)

Few men have contributed to as many fields in science as did Franz Cornelius Donders. He was a forerunner of Charles Darwin in evolutionary theory; his works paralleled those of Helmholtz in physics; and his classic description of the anomalies of accommodation and refraction of the human eye stamped him as one of the greatest clinical investigators in the field of ophthalmology.

He was born in Tilburg, North Brabant, in the Netherlands on the 27th of May, 1818. He was the only boy in the family and followed eight girls. His father was an unbusiness-like man whose interests lay in music, chemistry and literature, and who died of so-called "congestion of the brain" soon after the birth of his son. As a result there was little money available for Franz's education.

It is recorded that Franz was a precocious child and would be set upon a table in the local "pub" and given half-pennies for doing mental arithmetic before the marvelling locals. Even as a child he was paymaster to a large concern nearby. His mother wrote of this: "Imagine the little boy with dark eyes peeping out of the black locks, sitting behind the desk to give the coins to the big workmen!" Another of his duties was the regulation of the city clock. By the age of eleven, "Master Franz," as he was called, was employed as a salaried tutor at the school he attended.

Proceeding to the seminaries at Tilburg and Boxmeer, he learned to converse in French, Latin, Greek and English. He also took up the violin. At one stage he was contemplating entering the ministry, but gave this up for medicine, from which calling he never looked back, despite the difficulties he faced financially and the unsettled political situation brought about by Belgium's struggle to break away from Holland.

At age seventeen, Donders entered upon his medical course at the University of Utrecht, being attached as a pupil at the Military Hospital. In later years he wrote retrospectively of this period:

"Indescribable was the impression made upon me here by the chemical lectures and experiments of Nicolas de Fremery. When for the first time I mastered the notion that all that exists, in its infinite variety, is composed of a relatively small number of elements, which in certain proportions unite and reunite, it seemed to me as if, with the creation of the elements, the whole of nature had been given, and my imagination worked this out in its own way. Later, I became especially interested in physiology."

Because Donders finished his course before he was old enough to graduate at Utrecht, he transferred to the University of Leyden where he presented his graduation thesis: "Dissertatio inauguralis sistens observationes anatomico-pathologicas de centro nervoso." This thesis, based on original work, Donders presented in 1840, at the age of twenty-two. It was well received by his elders and Donders became a marked man. When he commenced his military service, therefore, it was not long before the Director General of the Dutch Medical Services singled him out for special duties. By dint of his unceasing labour in the hospital wards and post-mortem rooms at Flushing and at The Hague, he achieved the chair in anatomy, physiology and histology in the re-organized

Military Medical School, at the age of twenty-four. It is sobering to think of the teaching duties which he had to assume, *viz:* eighteen lectures per week for forty-six weeks each year! Only one who had been a tutor since the age of eleven could handle such a load.

At the age of twenty-six he began to turn over in his mind the possibility that there was a law of the conservation of energy in all of Nature. (It is interesting that another future ophthalmologist, Helmholtz, at age twenty-six, was to enunciate his famous theory on this subject.) Early in 1845, Donders read his paper to the Society of Sciences in Utrecht, on "A glance at the change of matter of epitellurian life as the source of proper heat of plants and animals."

His undergraduate musings in the field of chemistry recurred as he wrote: "All working in Nature, all life on earth, rests on the change of the elements from which it is formed, but side by side with this change of matter stands a change of forces. Both are inseparably bound up together."

"No one molecule of matter can be destroyed, but neither can a minimum of Energy. . . . Determinate quantities of movement, heat, light, electricity, magnetism, and nervous force respond to each other, and can pass from one into the other. . . . There is therefore a sum of energy, just as much as there is a sum of matter; both are proportionate to each other, both remain always the same."

On becoming Professor Extraordinary at the University of Utrecht in 1847, Donders gave an inaugural address on "The Harmony of Animal Life, a Manifestation of Laws." He shows clearly in this discourse how truly he was a forerunner of Charles Darwin, whom he later came to know and whom he visited at Down. Briefly, Donders stated the laws to be those of habit, exercise and inheritance. He wrote: "Already some light dawns in science on the causes of the phenomena we referred to, the laws of habit and of exercise; and thus, ascending from cause to cause, without ever losing ourselves in dreams about the purpose, we approach, slowly it is true, but with firm step, the ideal point of view, according to which all the phenomena of nature will be seen proceeding from the attribute of the elements and elementary forces. And if once by an All-wise Omnipotence these elements and forces have been created for a predetermined purpose, and if the conditions of the whole future have been enshrined in their attributes, then, also, not a single drop of blood flows without purpose through our veins, but it is a purpose which lies outside the science of nature."

Donders wrote to Darwin in 1871 about the state of the subject in the year 1847—"I tried to show how the infinite harmonical relations, on the one hand between animals and surrounding nature, on the other hand between the different parts and organs of every organism, are to be deduced from the laws of adaptation by habitude and by exercise, and from the laws of transmission . . . but still was not aware of the influence of natural selection, your great and immortal discovery, the mighty factor, which alone allowed (one) to give a full and special demonstration of the theory of descent."

Donders' work in physiological optics developed, and he undertook enough clinical practice in this field to eke out a living for his growing family. He was given a temporary hospital in which to work, and did not tell the University of Utrecht until years later that this had determined him to remain there at the moment that the entire medical faculty at Bonn had invited him to fill Helmholtz's chair. He developed his practice and research to such a degree that in 1864 he was able to encompass the whole of one of the principal fields of ophthalmology in his classical work, "On the Anomalies of Accommodation and Refraction of the Eye, with a Preliminary Essay on Physiological Dioptrics." Donders went on to investigate pitch in vowel sounds, "reaction time," "Muscular Work and Development of Heat in relation to the Necessary Elements of Food," "The Influence of the Vagus Nerve on the Cardiac Movements," and "The Chemical Phenomena of Respiration."

Snellen, his pupil, succeeded him in the hospital and Donders was given the chair of physiology in the University. There, he wrote on colour sense and colour blindness, and personally examined without remuneration many of the railway personnel of Holland in the interests of his campaign for safety on railroads and at sea. He took on many public duties and became Rector of his University.

On his retirement in May of 1888, the Royal Society of

London sent as its representatives to the Jubilee Celebration, Joseph Lister, Jonathan Hutchinson and Hughlings Jackson, surely a tribute to any man. A very large subscription was taken up in his honour, and at his request was used to found a series of travelling fellowships for work in physiology and ophthalmology. He died within a year of this great testimonial.

Adolf Kussmaul (1822-1902)

The noisy, gasping respiration of a diabetic patient in coma is known to medical students still as "Kussmaul's air hunger," having been described in 1874 by a very remarkable German physician. Kussmaul came from a medical family in Karlsruhe and graduated in medicine at Heidelberg at the age of twenty-three. While an undergraduate he became interested in the problem of the color of the pupil in the human eye, especially the variations noted in patients with glaucoma. He noted that the darkness of the pupil merely reflected the lack of light within the globe. By every means Kussmaul tried to illuminate the interior of the eye, as by immersing it in water, whereupon the vessels of the retina became visible. The ophthalmoscope which he designed failed to meet the requirements, but the determination displayed and the clarification of the problem achieved, mark Kussmaul as a true forerunner of Helmholtz in ophthalmology. Kussmaul's student work won for him the Karl Fredrick Gold Medal which was awarded at the re-dedication ceremonies of the University of Heidelberg.

After graduation in 1845 Kussmaul served as an army doctor and general practitioner for several years until he was struck down with a disease resembling poliomyelitis, which affected his legs. He returned to academic life at Wurzburg where the youthful Virchow was revolutionizing pathology. Thereafter Kussmaul served in the chair of medicine at Heidelberg, Erlangen, Freiburg and Strasbourg. He was the first to describe progressive bulbar palsy, periarteritis nodosa, and the visual inspection of the oesophagus and stomach by a lighted tube.

Kussmaul wrote his *Recollections of Youth by an old physician* in 1899, and from it one may get an unforgettable impression of the changes which occurred over the period of Kussmaul's long and useful life. Osler wrote of Kussmaul:

How true sometimes is the paradox of the Gospel that to save his life a man must lose it! . . . In that best of all medical autobiographies . . . Kussmaul tells the story of his student days and of the happy beginning of a busy life as district physician in the Black Forest—plenty of work, good health, and a happy home with wife and children. Then the overwhelming disaster—sudden paraplegia, a long struggle in adverse circumstances, and a final Victory wrought out of the very elements of defeat.

Hermann Von Helmholtz (1821-1894)

Hermann Ludwig Ferdinand von Helmholtz was born at Potsdam, Germany, on August 21, 1821. His father was a teacher of philosophy and philology in the Gymnasium and was a man widely respected for his ability and integrity. His mother was the daughter of an artillery officer from Hanover, named Penn, a descendent of William Penn, the founder of Pennsylvania.

Growing up as a sickly child and spending much time in bed, Helmholtz learned to read early and he read very widely. With the wooden blocks which his parents provided for him he began to develop rudimentary geometric skills. Though he had early difficulty with languages, he was able by the age of eight, to read Homer, and by the age of twelve he was reading Arabic fables.

His health improving, he attended the Gymnasium in Potsdam, where he astonished his teachers with his knowledge of Geometry. Among his fellow students was Du Bois Reymond, later to distinguish himself in the field of electrophysiology. Helmholtz soon became an avid nature observer and savoured the full range of his father's excellent library. While his classmates in the Gymnasium studied classics he, by subterfuge, drew many diagrams of the pathway of light through the lenses of telescopes. Using some old botanists' magnifying glasses, he set up a great variety of optical systems for his own diversion.

Helmholtz's father wished him to study medicine because there were three other children to think about in the family and some economic independence was thought essential. Helmholtz himself wanted to do physics but once admitted to the Royal Medical-Chirurgical Friedrich-Wilhelm Institute in Berlin, he took up his studies with great enthusiasm. The rector of the Gymnasium in Potsdam provided him with the following certificate of entrance to University: "His exceptionally calm and reserved disposition is combined with great intellectual enthusiasm. In it we recognize an excellent combination of clear and prudent understanding and deep good nature. His manners bear witness to a carefully preserved, exceptionally pure, and genuine childlike innocence. These peculiarities, along with the richness and power of his mental development give an agreeable and captivating impression, and justify the hope that such a ground-soil of intellectual life will only bring forth the best of fruits."

In return for the Army subsidy which he was receiving at the University of Berlin, the agreement was that Helmholtz, along with the other subsidized graduates, would return to the Army for service. At the University of Berlin, Helmholtz came under the all-pervading influence of one of the greatest physiologists of all time, Johannes Müller. Helmholtz served him as a student demonstrator, as did such future giants as Du Bois Reymond, Brucke, and Rudolf Virchow. Under the influence of Johannes Müller and Gustav Magnus, the Professor of Physics, a great impetus to investigation was imparted to these young men. The medical course was broadly conceived and was basic enough to serve as a foundation for three brilliant careers in quite separate parts of the scientific field.

The stimulating atmosphere which Helmholtz found is best described in his own words: "My own original inclination was towards physics; external circumstances obliged me to commence the study of medicine. It had, however, been the custom of a former time to combine the study of medicine with that of the natural sciences and, whatever in this was compulsory, I must consider fortunate; not merely that I entered medicine at a time in which anyone who was even moderately at home in physical considerations found virgin field for cultivation, but I consider the study of medicine to have been that training which preached more impressively and more convincingly than any other could have done, the everlasting principles of all scientific work; principles which are so simple and yet are ever forgotten; so clear and yet always so hidden by a deceptive veil."

Helmholtz's mathematics were entirely self taught. He never studied under any great mathematician and yet, as we shall see later, he was very much at home in this subject, thanks to his excellent grounding.

The University of Berlin in common with many Universities of Europe of the time had that most admirable requirement of a dissertation or thesis which a candidate for the medical degree was obliged to present upon graduation. Ever since the discovery by Ehrenberg, in 1833, of nerve cells, Helmholtz had been anxious to explore these building blocks of the nervous system. In his final year of medicine, he suffered an attack of typhus fever and, in true Army fashion, he was hospitalized without expense, and he was thus able to save up a small sum of money. With this he bought the microscope which he used to make the great discovery embodied in his thesis. What Helmholtz discovered—the fact that the nerve cells were actually connected with the peripheral nerves—seems elementary to us today. However, it is to Helmholtz that we owe the proof, given with his primitive compound microscope, that the "corpuscles" in the ganglia of leeches and crabs, were actually the origin of the nerve fibres. He immediately proceeded with the generalization that the axis cylinder proceeds from the axon hillock or pole of the nerve cell and is continued out into the periphery as the nerve fibre.

Just before he completed his undergraduate work, he read a paper on venous tumours before the Institute for the Education of Army Surgeons. Thereafter Helmholtz published several papers annually until his death in 1894, a total of two hundred seventeen papers and books.

In 1842, Helmholtz graduated from Medical School and served his year as an assistant physician in La Charité Hospital in Berlin. In 1843, he became assistant surgeon to the Red Hussars Regiment. The great Alexander von Humboldt had Helmholtz relieved of some of his military duties at Potsdam so that he could become assistant to the anatomical museum, lecturer on anatomy to the Academy of Arts, and extraordinary Professor of Physiology to the Albert University!

Thus began his great work on the heat of contraction of muscles. He measured accurately also the heat lost from the body through expiration and evaporation from the skin. He devised the "Myograph" or the muscle writer, to measure what Thomas

"The history of medicine . . . can claim a very special interest in the history of the development of human thought, for no other history is better adapted to demonstrate that a correct criticism of the sources of our knowledge is practically one of the most important duties of true philosophy."

—Helmholtz.

"The value of a man is not measured by the truth he possesses, but rather by his sincere effort to discover truth. For it is not through possession of truth, but much more by search for it that his powers are widened, those powers which conduce to evergrowing perfection."

—Lessing.

Young had always called for, the exact time relations of muscle activity.

It was while library assistant in the Frederick Wilhelm Institute that Helmholtz filled his "idle moments" by reading the chief mathematical works of the eighteenth century. At the age of twenty-six he wrote his essay on "The conservation of energy," which he read before the Physical Society of Berlin. Most of the members of the Society were openly hostile to the ideas which he expressed in his paper. However, George Ernst Reimer, the publisher, was so impressed with the author that he put the essay in print and even paid for it himself. Helmholtz's superior officers in the German Army were so impressed that they relieved him of most of his military duties and gave him still more time for research. It is typical of Helmholtz that he never ceased to praise the Heilbronn general practitioner, Robert Mayer, who had independently and, at an earlier date, demonstrated the first law of thermodynamics—that all types of energy are transformable but indestructible. Mayer's demonstration applied only to the physiological sphere. Helmholtz applied it as a generalization to all spheres of experience. What better place than an army barracks in which to write on the conservation of energy!

At the age of twenty-nine, Helmholtz was appointed to the chair of Physiology at Königsberg; at the age of thirty-five to the chair in Bonn; at the age of thirty-eight to Heidelberg and at the age of fifty he was called to the chair of Physics in Berlin, where he served until his death in 1894.

In 1850, a mere ten years after Johannes Müller stated his opinion that the speed of transmission of the nerve impulse could never be measured, Helmholtz succeeded in measuring it. In 1851, Helmholtz invented the ophthalmoscope for which contribution alone humanity should remember him. Bearing upon the two discoveries above mentioned, Helmholtz said, "A teacher in a University is subject to excellent discipline, in that he is obliged each year, not only to give at least an outline of the whole of his science, but also to convince and satisfy the clear heads among his hearers, some of whom will be the great men of the next generation. This necessity was most beneficial to myself. In preparing my lectures, I was led to devise a method of measuring the velocity of the nerve impulse and also the conception of the ophthalmoscope." Charles Babbage in England, the great mathematician who built cogwheel calculators almost as complex as the present electronic computors, showed the British ophthalmologist, Wharton Jones, how to use a small silvered mirror to reflect light into the eye, the eye being observed through a small central peephole. The application of a lens system to Babbage's suggested instrument might well have established the priority of the British scientist, but nothing ever came of it. When in December 1850, Helmholtz gave his first report of his instrument, before the Berlin Physical Society, the response was immediate and tumultuous.

In the succeeding years Helmholtz did pioneering work in the fields of acoustics, vision, dynamics, convection, and electrical energy, and he even regarded chemical atoms as basically electrical entities. It is little wonder that in his laboratory, his pupil Hertz discovered the waves which led eventually to wireless communication. Helmholtz published his great *Handbook of Physiological Optics*, which was produced from the years 1856-1867 and has become a classic. He revived Thomas Young's theory of colour vision and thought of it as a very specialized application of Johannes Müller's law of specific nerve energies.

Helmholtz was interested in all natural phenomena and wrote on such diverse subjects as cloud formations and the effect of wind on the length of waves in the sea. He was interested also in the study of glaciers. He even wrote a paper on hayfever and, in his own case, its apparent control by the application of a dilute solution of quinine sulphate to the nasal mucous membrane.

He loved to play Bach on the grand piano given to him by the Steinway Company of New York in recognition of his services to music. Above all, Helmholtz liked to be regarded as a teacher. As a writer in the *Edinburgh Medical Journal* for 1859 said, "He treats every subject with which he is engaged with a most masterly and philosophical spirit and investigates all things independently for himself, never resting content with the tradition of the early physiologists." This common denominator runs through the lives of many in this volume.

Thirty-five years after graduating from the Army Medical Institute in Berlin, he returned to give what was one of his greatest lectures, "Thought in medicine." Here he summed up his philosophy of medical discovery and medical change. Speaking in the same hall in which he had reported his early student papers he said: "Medicine was once the intellectual home in which I grew up; and even the emigrant best understands and is best understood by his native land."

The most succinct obituary notice on Helmholtz appeared soon after his death in London's famous *Punch:*

> "What matters titles, Helmholtz is a name,
> That challenges alone the award of fame.
> When Emperors, Kings, Pretenders, shadows all,
> Leave not a dust trace on our whirling ball
> Thy work, O grave-eyed Searcher, shall endure,
> Unmarred by faction, from low passion pure."

PLATE 9

(a) Hermann von Helmholtz (1821-1894) as a young man. Courtesy of the Bettmann Archive, New York.

(b) Drawings of three models of Galileo's *pulsilogia* designed while he was a student of medicine.

(c) Young's arrangement of the last line of the Rosetta Stone. From: Oldham, Frank: *Thomas Young, F.R.S., Philosopher and Physician,* 1933. Courtesy of the author and of Edward Arnold and Co., London.

(d) Thomas Young, F.R.S. (1773-1829). Portrait by Sir Thomas Lawrence. From: Oldham, Frank: *Thomas Young, F.R.S., Philosopher and Physician,* 1933. Courtesy of the author and of Edward Arnold and Co., London.

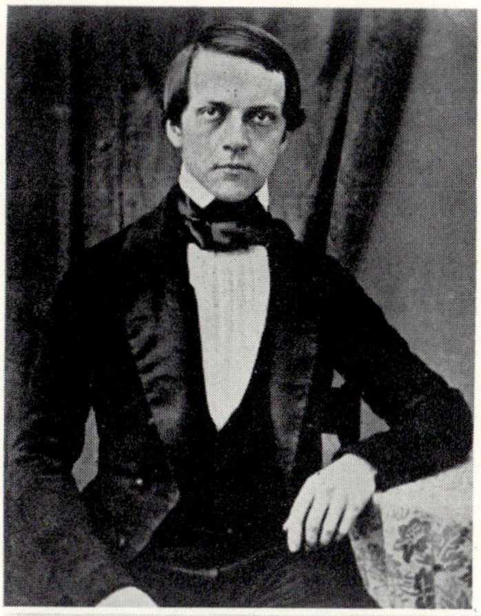

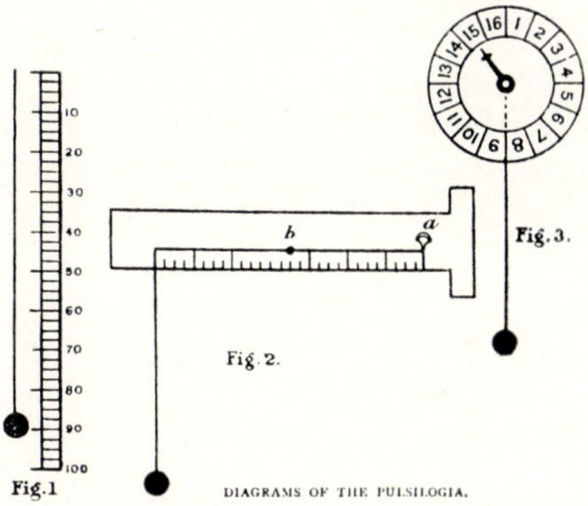

DIAGRAMS OF THE PULSILOGIA.

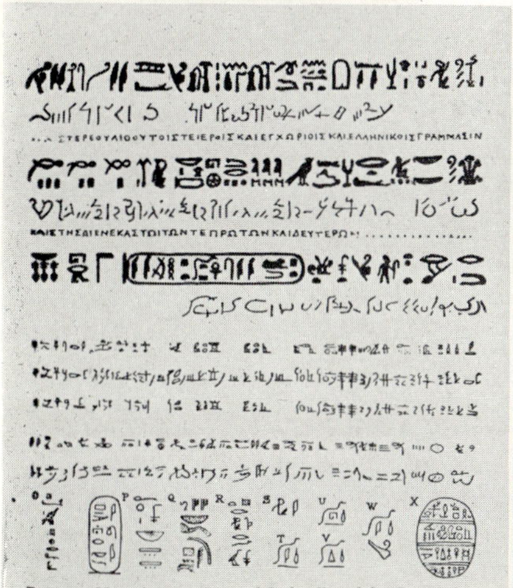

FIG. 10.—Young's arrangement of the last line of the Rosetta Stone.

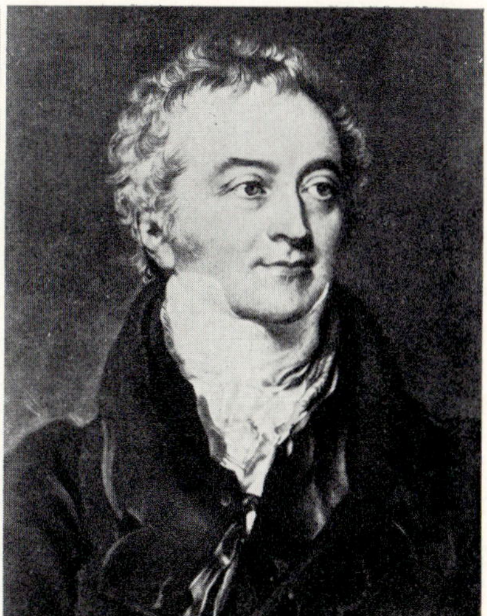

←

Chapter XII

Conclusions

"And some seed fell on the good ground and grew and brought forth fruit a hundred fold."

THE FOREGOING CHAPTERS have shown nothing if not the kaleidoscopic nature of life as it has been lived by students and physicians over the past four hundred years. And yet it is basically a study in growth of men and of their ideas, with much depending on the seed, the soil, the nourishment provided, the losses and wastage, and the weather at harvest time. If we are good farmers we may profit by the experience condensed into these chapters.

The seed was obviously the critical factor throughout. Without it there would be nothing to discuss. These students obviously had gray matter. Some feel that we are not getting the available gray matter in our population within hailing distance of our universities, and they convincingly quote the National Science Foundation of the United States to the effect that only one quarter of the top students, academically, who graduate from American high schools, ever reach university. A study of *why* this is so is imperative.

Some may ask: "If we had the remaining three-quarters of the brightest high school graduates within our universities would we have any more student discoverers? Do we not, in some institutions, tend to have a rigid set of rewards and blessings heavily inclined towards the spectacular performer in the classroom?" As James Kendall has remarked in his delightful book, *Young Chemists and Great Discoveries*, the great Leipzig chemist, Wilhelm Ostwald, used to say that his pupils who later became famous contributors were not those at the head of their classes, but were those who had not been satisfied with what had been given out routinely in the classroom. The student contributors in the present volume could be said to have had a constructive curiosity. It is of the type exhibited by the youthful Michael Faraday—son of a blacksmith and apprenticed to a bookbinder, whose early education consisted in the reading of the volumes which he was binding. This constructive curiosity may be seen in the lives of such physician botanists as Valerius Cordus, Haller, Linnaeus, Garden, Schleiden and Withering, such physician geologists as Bright, Stensen and Jenner, or such ornithologists as T. S. Roberts, the Minnesota pediatrician, and Max Peet, the Michigan neurosurgeon. Some educators feel that with the hubbub of modern university campuses some of the best seed never even falls to the ground, so diverse are the currents of air which sweep over our students and so powerful are the tribal organizations which mold them socially. The passive rôle of the student is taken for granted in so many colleges that the student who seeks new answers may be a cause for official alarm. Just as college athletics have become spectator sports instead of participant sports, so medical education has become spectator-centered, with participation by students glossed over.

It may be remarked that some of the seed may be rather odd in appearance or behavior but this is patently irrelevant to the main matter of the scientific contribution to be made. Semmelweis, Horsley, Blake and Carrion were no ordinary men, to mention only a few of our student group, but they advanced humanity—just as the brilliant but neurotic chemist, Carothers, did with his development of nylon.

Another question may be asked: "Was fame the spur in the students discussed in this volume?" It is inconceivable that Semmelweis lived only for the day when his researches on tartar

"Nobody knows how the kindling flame of life and power leaps from one life to another. What is the magic quality in a person which instantly awakens faith? You listen to a hundred persons unmoved and unchanged; you hear a few quiet words from the man with the kindling torch and you suddenly discover what life means for you forever more, and you become forthwith another man, carrying perhaps, your own torch."

—RUFUS JONES.

"From my point of view there is only one intellectual infection of any permanent value to the medical student—the scientific spirit and outlook and attitude of mind, which he gets, often unconsciously from his teachers and fellows. If good, it leavens his life work. That he may be steeped in it and be at the same time thoroughly practical is the experience of scores of teachers and scores of pupils, of men of the type of Bowman and Paget. The practical man (whom Mr. C-G. has lauded) was well defined by a general practitioner in my company a few moments ago as one who never learns anything after leaving his hospital. I should be grievous sorry to have any student in whom I was interested come under the influence of a man who in these days could say that 'scientific education may be excellent as an ideal but I doubt if it materially assists the average practitioner in the treatment of disease.' Mr. G. represents a type—the men who jeered at Harvey, scoffed at Pasteur and scorned Lister—the carpenters in surgery and the pill-mongers in medicine, without vision beyond the bench or the counter. The tragedy is that the type persists."

—WILLIAM OSLER (1913).

emetic in experimental pneumonia would make him famous, though it was the beginning of his interest in infection. Lister, gazing through his microscope at the muscles of the iris, was not consciously launching his crusade against sepsis, though the talents which he thus developed at the microscope led him there. William Harvey, assisting in the researches of his teacher Fabricius, in Padua, little dreamed that he would gather "fame" in the field of the circulation of the blood, or that he would, as a result, lose much of his practice in England.

This brings us to the question of "the soil." We have seen that in the laboratory of William Sharpey at University College, London, Lister, Huxley and James Blake made their early contributions. In Johannes Müller's laboratory, in Berlin, Remak, Helmholtz and Gruby first put their hands to research. Carl Ludwig taught the techniques of investigation to Henry Bowditch, who, in turn, encouraged the student Walter Cannon to apply x-rays to the movements of the gut in animals in his Boston laboratory. In modern times the laboratories of Sir Henry Dale and Sir Charles Sherrington became veritable powerhouses from which hundreds of researchers received their initial stimulus. Sympathetic teachers have done much to encourage discovery.

Sir Geoffrey Jefferson in his review of some British pioneers in neurology comments on students who have been, reciprocally, great fertilizers of their teachers' imaginations. He tells of James Ross (1837-1892) holding a bedside clinic at the Manchester Royal Infirmary, on the subject of pleurisy in that part of the lung which touches the diaphragm, sometimes causing a sharp pain in the tip of the shoulder. Ross has recorded that: "In observing a case of pleurisy a few days ago and casting about for an explanation, one of the students suggested that, considering the connections of the phrenic, the pain might be caused by that nerve." This student, without knowing it, opened up one of the most interesting fields in medicine, that of "referred pain." Purkinje was famous for allowing students to announce in papers which they were writing discoveries which he had made.

Students' medical societies and students' medical libraries have had a great catalytic effect in this field. Sir William Bowman, whose name remains attached to structures in the eye and the

"When I was a boy I wanted to know about the clouds and the grasses, and why the leaves changed colour in the autumn; I watched the ants, bees, birds, tadpoles and cadis worms; I pestered people with questions about what nobody knew or cared anything about."

—John Hunter.

"It were disgraceful, therefore, did we take the reports of others upon trust, and go on coining crude problems out of these, and on them hanging knotty and captious and petty disputations. Nature herself is to be addressed; the paths she shows us are to be boldly trodden; for thus, and whilst we consult our proper senses . . . shall we penetrate at length into the heart of her mystery."

—William Harvey.

". . . For many reasons it is desirable that a medical student be conducted early in his career to the front line trenches of medical and physiological discovery. Let him realize that men as young as himself have made important contributions: that de Graaf at 23 years of age devised the first pancreatic fistula; that Helmholtz at 24 measured for the first time the heat production of frog muscle; that Johannes Muller at 25 had enunciated the principles of specific nerve energies. Let him discover that simple facts were once hidden in a fog of faulty observation and faulty reasoning, and that it was sometimes the enquiring minds of students like himself that made matters clear."

—John Farquhar Fulton.

kidney, read papers at his student society on haemorrhage, influenza and paraplegia. William Withering as an undergraduate at Edinburgh read two papers to his student society on dropsy, little realizing that as a practitioner in Shropshire he would soon learn from "Old Mother Hutton" of the value of foxglove in the treatment of this disease. A good library and a sympathetic librarian are essential to the development of student contributors. Thanks to the goal set by John Shaw Billings as an undergraduate, all students today have access to the world's medical literature through indices and current lists of the contents of journals, and through microfilms and photostats from the Armed Forces Medical Library in Washington, D. C.

The choice of a target has helped some to contribute where there was no hospitable soil for the germination of ideas. John Hunter set himself to study inflammation when he was an almost illiterate student; his great work on this subject was published in the last year of his life! (It is related that Abraham Lincoln, floating down the Mississippi on a river barge, at the age of nineteen, picked out his target—and held to it until the slaves were freed.) Semmelweis marked out his target as he took special work in obstetrics a few months before he graduated. On seeing the crude barbers doing the dissecting in Paris, Vesalius decided to wrest the scalpel from them, and to describe in his book the true structure of the human body. Carrion, like an arrow, went straight to the heart of Oroya fever and died in the process. These students lacked the guidance of teachers, and indeed made their contributions despite deep-rooted opposition.

The nourishment of the seed in the soil has taken some strange forms historically; the means of support were sometimes pitiful in the extreme. Cotugno lived on radishes and bread and the charity of a hospital for incurables in Italy. Billings lived on a diet consisting, according to Weir Mitchell, of nothing but eggs and milk and the charity of a pioneer hospital in Ohio. Others served in assistantships or as demonstrators, such as Christopher Wren, who, after serving Harvey's pupil Sir Charles Scarborough from age 14 to 17 as a dissector at Surgeons' Hall in London, sought to pay his way through Oxford University by working for Thomas Willis, whose arterial "circle" in the base of the brain he was to illustrate in this capacity. Jean Fernel, and the dejected playwrights Claude Bernard and Brown-Séquard in Paris, lived on their earnings as tutors while pursuing medicine.

The time lost to study in some of these pursuits is discussed by Sir Weldon Dalrymple-Champneys in his recent paper, "The medical student through the ages," read before the Royal Society of Medicine in London in 1955. He quotes the complaint of a poor student at Bologna in the fifteenth century: "The time I should spend at lectures and in study I am driven to waste in begging from door to door, crying scores and scores of times, 'Charity, charity, dear masters,' and getting the answer 'Begone, and God be with you.' I appeal both to ecclesiastics and laymen, and am mostly driven from the door, or perchance one may say 'Wait a bit,' when I get a dirty scrap of bread which a dog would reject, or I may get fusty beans, bits of skin or gristle, or sour wine."

Before leaving this aspect of the subject, tribute should be paid to the military agencies which subsidized such medical students as Helmholtz, Donders and Pavlov, to name only a few. At a later stage in his career Billings was to have the blessing and financial support of General Barnes in the development of the Surgeon General's Library. What better use were residual canteen funds ever put to after a bitter war? The tradition of subsidizing medical student researchers is kept alive today by the Royal Canadian Air Force, which remembers with reason, the contributions made in World War II by Sir Frederick Banting's former "summer research" students in medicine.

Wastage may result from poor methods of tilling the soil, and against this evil the best seed is not proof. Charles Robert Darwin (1809-82) was lost to medicine because of the teaching he encountered, as we shall see. His interest in variation in species dates from his early childhood when he told an unsuspecting eight-year old playmate that he could develop any color in primroses by merely watering them with colored solutions! The truth proved to be stranger than even this fiction. He went to study medicine at the University of Edinburgh where his brother was completing his training. Of his own experiences there, Charles wrote:

The instruction at Edinburgh was altogether by lectures, and these were intolerably dull, with the exception of those on chemistry by Hope.

Dr. Monro (tertius) made his lectures as dull as he was himself, and the subject disgusted me. It has proved one of the greatest evils in my life that I was not urged to practise dissection, for I should soon have got over my disgust; and the practice would have been invaluable for all my future work. This has been an irremediable evil, as well as my incapacity to draw. I also attended regularly the clinical wards in the hospital. . . . I cannot understand why this part of my medical course did not interest me in a greater degree; for during the summer before coming to Edinburgh I began attending some of the poor people, chiefly children and women in Shrewsbury. I wrote down as full an account as I could of the case with all the symptoms, and read them aloud to my father, who suggested further enquiries and advised me what medicines to give, which I made up myself. At one time I had at least a dozen patients, and I felt keen interest in the work.

. . . I made one interesting little discovery, and read, about the beginning of the year 1826, a short paper on the subject before the Plinian Society. This was that the so-called ova of Flustra had the power of independent movement by means of cilia, and were in fact larvae. In another short paper I showed that the little globular bodies which had been supposed to be the young state of fucus loreus were the egg-cases of the wormlike Pontobdella muricata.

Darwin left Edinburgh in disgust and went to Cambridge where he took his B.A. degree in 1831. He joined Captain Fitz-Roy of *The Beagle*, as naturalist, unpaid, for the five-year circumnavigation of the globe. Twenty-three years after his return he published his *Origin of Species*. Darwin's loss to medicine may be counted a tragedy, so great were his powers of observation and generalization.

The harvest "weather" has varied considerably for our group of contributors. Einthoven's work was accepted from the first and he lived to see the greatest demonstrations of affectionate homage. But the unorthodoxy implied in searching for new truths, and in replacing old ideas with new, has usually collided with orthodoxy in some guise or other. Wilfred Trotter used to say that the mind welcomes a new idea about as graciously as the body welcomes a foreign protein! As we have seen Harvey lost a large part of his practice. George Sarton has remarked on the tactics

"He who ceases to try to do better ceases to do well."

—OLIVER CROMWELL.

"Medicine is a science which hath been more professed than laboured, and yet more laboured than advanced, the labour having been more in a circle than in progression."

—LORD BACON.

"Youth, however eclipsed for a season, is undoubtedly the proper, permanent and genuine condition of man."

—NATHANIEL HAWTHORNE.

"Greater even than the greatest discovery is to keep open the way to future discoveries."

—J. J. ABEL (1915).

of his critics; at first they said his "facts" were not true; then, in retreat, they argued that they were already well-known! Vesalius was pilloried by the "practical men," whom he reviled as being fit only to prescribe for the bowels. His contemporary, Servetus, was burned at the stake by John Calvin who fancied himself divinely guided and who would brook no rival views on theology even when mixed with the discovery of the circulation of the blood through the lungs. Similarly, Morton's ether anaesthesia was attacked by some clerics whose unctuous rectitude was exceeded only by their ignorance. Semmelweis was turned out of the General Hospital in Vienna, as was Freud forty years later. Stensen was attacked by his teacher Blasius, and Galileo was eventually imprisoned.

And finally we come to the future and what it holds, or can hold, for the young minds passing through our medical schools. We are all conscious of the need for prescribed courses for men and women who will one day care for the sick. There is no substitute for that central core of factual knowledge, but, as Alan Gregg has remarked, the mistakes in medicine are not made by the men who don't know, but by the men who don't care. By overloading our undergraduates with a phenomenal amount of detail in some subjects we obscure the person in bed, and probably manufacture "men who don't care." Over and above "the legal minimum" of instruction, however, we face the question of how best to develop the enquiring mind, for this mind surely is the patient's greatest guarantee of good diagnosis and rational treatment. It is, at the same time, the critical factor in discovery and progress in medical science.

We must, then, encourage enquiring minds in medicine. Harvey Cushing's criticism of medical education was that it proceeded in convoy fashion, the speed of the fleet being measured by the speed of the slowest ship. He would agree with Fuller's sentiments expressed in 1639 in his *Holy Warre*—"Good is not good when proceeding from them from whom farre better is expected." Do we, in fact, expect enough from our brighter students? Do we challenge them to begin educating themselves or do we force them to become cynical young onlookers?

What sort of opportunity should be given to "dangerous

young infidels" on their way through medical school? The answer can be found in the imagination displayed by Richard Bright over a century ago, in his study of kidney disease and its relation to high blood pressure. In 1842 he was granted by the Governors of Guy's Hospital the use of two wards for a period of six months. The room between the two wards was "fitted up entirely to our purpose" as a laboratory. This constituted the first Clinical Investigation Unit in Britain. For manpower in this research endeavour he pressed into service four "clinicals" whom, he said, he "selected from the more advanced pupils, who have distinguished themselves by their diligence and ability in reporting in the general wards." Thus Tweedie, Barlow and Reese studied the urines of 269 cases of nephritis who passed through the wards in six months, and George Robinson examined microscopically the kidneys of all fatal cases. With this array of talent the nephritic fortress was reduced in six months. There were no application forms in eighteen copies, no security clearances, no public relations officers—just imagination backed by the hard work of dedicated students.

If the history summarized in these pages helps us, students and teachers alike, to be more imaginative investigators of Nature, it will have been well worth the writing.

Bibliography

Books of General Reference

Bast, T. H.: *The Life and Times of Adolf Kussmaul.* New York, Hoeber, 1926.

Camac, C. N. B., (coll.).: *Epoch-making Contributions to Medicine, Surgery and the Allied Sciences.* Philadelphia and London. W. B. Saunders Company, 1909. (435 pp.)

Camac, C. N. B.: *Imhotep to Harvey.* New York, Hoeber, 1931. (324 pp.)

Cannon, W. B.: *The Way of an Investigator.* New York, W. W. Norton Co., 1945. (229 pp.)

Castiglioni, A.: *A History of Medicine.* (2nd ed.). New York, Knopf, 1947.

Conant, J. B.: *On Understanding Science. An historical approach.* New Haven, Yale University Press, 1947. (146 pp.)

Dale, Sir Henry H.: *An Autumn Gleaning.* London, Pergamon Press, 1954. (225 pp.)

Flexner, J. T.: *Doctors on Horseback—Pioneers of American Medicine.* New York, Viking, 1937. (370 pp.)

Foster, Sir Michael: *Lectures on the History of Physiology.* Cambridge, University Press, 1924. (306 pp.)

Garrison, Fielding H.: *An Introduction to the History of Medicine,* (4th ed.). Philadelphia and London, W. B. Saunders Company, 1929.

Griffith, E. F.: *Doctors by Themselves.* London, Cassell, 1951. (614 pp.)

Hale-White, Sir W.: *Great Doctors of the Nineteenth Century.* London, Arnold, 1935.

Haymaker, Webb: *Founders of Neurology.* Springfield, Thomas, 1953. (479 pp.)

Hemmeter, John C.: *Master Minds in Medicine.* New York, Medical Life Press, 1927.

Kelly, E. C.: *Encyclopedia of Medical Sources.* Baltimore, Williams-Wilkins, 1948. (476 pp.)

Long, Esmond R.: *Selected Readings in Pathology.* Springfield, Thomas, 1929.

Major, Ralph H.: *Classic Descriptions of Disease.* Springfield, Thomas, 1932. (630 pp.)

Meisen, V. (ed.).: *Prominent Danish Scientists Through the Ages with Facsimiles from Their Works.* Copenhagen, Levin & Munksgaard, 1932. (195 pp.)

Monro, T. K.: *The Physician as Man of Letters, Science and Action,* (2nd ed.). Edinburgh, Livingstone, 1951. (259 pp.)

Osler, Sir William: *The Evolution of Modern Medicine.* New Haven, Yale University Press, 1921.

Penfield, W. G. et al.: *Neurological Biographies and Addresses.* London, Oxford University Press, 1936. (pp. 178.)

Stevenson, Lloyd: *Sir Frederick Banting.* Toronto, Ryerson, 1946.

Woglom, W. H.: *Discoverers for Medicine.* New Haven, Yale University Press, 1949.

Anaesthesia

Cartwright, F. F.: *The English Pioneers of Anaesthesia.* Bristol, J. Wright and Sons, 1952.

Davy, Sir H.: *Collected Works,* Vol. 3. London, Smith, Elder and Co., 1839.

Fulton, J. F., Duveen, D., and Klickstein, H. S.: Antoine Laurent Lavoisier's Reflexions sur les Effets de l'Ether Vitriolique et de l'Ether Nitreux dans l'Economie Animale. *J. History Med., 8:*318-323, 1953.

Keys, Thomas E.: *The History of Surgical Anaesthesia.* New York, Shuman, 1945.

Leake, C. D.: Valerius Cordus and the discovery of ether. *Isis,* 7:14-24, 1925.

Paris, John A.: *The Life of Sir Humphry Davy.* London, Henry Colburn and Richard Bentley, 1831.

Young, Hugh H.: Long, the discoverer of anaesthesia, a presentation of his original documents. *Bull. Johns Hopkins Hosp., 8:*174-184, 1897.

Anatomy

Ball, J. M.: *Andreas Vesalius.* St. Louis, Med. Sci. Press, 1910.

Castiglioni, A.: Andreas Vesalius, Professor at the Medical School of Padua. *Bull. N.Y. Acad. Med., 19:*766-777, 1943.

Dobson, Jessie: Frederick Oldfield Ward. *J. Bone and Joint Surg., 31B:*596-599, 1949.

Dobson, Jessie: Frederick Augustus Dixey. *J. Bone and Joint Surg., 33B:*275-277, 1951.

Fisch, M. H.: "Vesalius and his book." *Bull. Med. Libr. Assn., 31:*208-221, 1943.

Harris, D. Fraser: Eminent Undergraduate Observers. *Medical Life, 32:*111-116, 1925.

Huxley, Julian: *T. H. Huxley's Diary of the Voyage of H. M. S. Rattlesnake.* New York, Doubleday, Doran, 1936.

Huxley, Leonard: *Life and Letters of Thomas Henry Huxley,* (3 vols.). New York, Macmillan Co., 1903, (2nd ed.).

Keith, Sir Arthur: *An Autobiography.* London, Watt, 1950.

Leeson, John R.: *Lister as I Knew him.* London, Baillière, Tindall & Cox, 1927.

Lister, Joseph: Observations on the contractile tissue of the iris. *Quart. J. Microsc. Sci., 1:*8-17, 1853.

Lister, Joseph: Observations on the Muscular Tissue of the Skin. *Quart. J. Microsc. Sci., 1:*262-268, 1853.

Montagu, M. F. Ashley: Vesalius and the Galenists, in *Science, Medicine, and History,* ed. E. A. Underwood. London, Oxford University Press, 1953, 2 vol.

Ramón y Cajal, S.: *Recollections of my life.* Translated by E. Horne Craigie. *Memoirs Amer. Philos. Soc., 8:*pts. 1 and 2, 1937.

Teller, J. D.: The Social Responsibility of a Scientist. *Education, 63:* 3-10, 1942.

Welch, Wm.: The Times of Vesalius, Contributions of Vesalius other than Anatomical. *Bull. Johns Hopkins Hosp., 26:*118-120, 1915.

Bibliographers

Billings, J. S.: The Surgical Treatment of Epilepsy. *Cincinnati Lancet & Observer,* n.s. *4:*334, 1861.

Billings, J. S.: The Medical College of Ohio before the war. *Cincinnati Lancet-Clinic, 20:*297-305, 1888.

Billings, J. S.: Mechanical methods used in compiling data of the eleventh U.S. Census; with an exhibition of a machine. *Proc. Amer. Assoc. Adv. Sc., 40:*407-409, 1891.

Chesney, A. M.: John Shaw Billings and the Johns Hopkins Medical School. *Bull. Inst. Hist. Med., 6:*271-286, 1938.

Cordasco, F.: *A Bibliography of Robert Watt, M.D.* New York, W. F. Kelleher, 1950.

Curran, J. A.: John Shaw Billings. Medical Genius of the 19th Century. Speech to Friends of the Armed Forces Medical Library, Washington, D.C. 23 October 1953.

Fulton, J. F.: *The Great Medical Bibliographers.* Philadelphia, University of Pennsylvania Press, 1951. (pp. 15, 107.)

Hume, E. E.: John Shaw Billings as an Army Officer. *Bull. Inst. Hist. Med., 6:*225-270, 1938.

Osler, W.: at the Memorial Meeting in honor of Dr. John Shaw Billings, April 25, 1913. *Bull. N.Y. Public Library, 17:*511-530, 1913.

Cardio-vascular System

Brock, R. C.: *The life and work of Astley Cooper.* Edinburgh, E. & S. Livingstone Ltd., 1952. (pp. 176.)

Dale, H. H.: Obituary Notice of Sir Thomas Lewis. *Brit. M.J., 1:*461, 1945.

del Rio-Hortega, P.: El Tercer elemento de los centros nerviosos. *Bol. Soc. espan. de biol., 9:*69, 1919.

Einthoven, W.: Elektrokardiogramms. *Arch. ges. Physiol., 99:*472-480, 1903.

Flack, Martin: Milroy Lectures. *Lancet, 2:*637, 693, 1921. Obituary Note. *Lancet, 2:*430, 510, 1931. *Brit. Med. J., 2:*402, 1931.

Foster, M.: *Lectures on the History of Physiology.* Cambridge, University Press, 1924. (pp. 306.)

Keith, Sir Arthur: *An Autobiography.* London, Watts, 1950.

Kershman, J.: Genesis of microglia in the human brain. *Arch. Neurol. & Psychiat., 41:*24-50, 1939.

Leake, C. D.: Translation: *Anatomical Studies on the Motion of the Heart and Blood,* by William Harvey, M.D. Springfield, Thomas, 1930. (150 pp.)

Lewis, Thomas: Observations on the functions of the spleen and other haemolymph glands. *J. Anat. & Physiol., 38:*144-157, 1904.

Lewis, Sir Thomas: Willem Einthoven, obituary notice. *Brit. M.J., 2:*664-665, 1927.

MacCallum, J. B.: Fresh Water Cladocera. *Univ. Toronto Quart., 1:* 104-112, 1895.

Idem.: On the histology and histogenesis of the heart muscle cell. *Anat. Anz., 13:*609-620, 1897.

Idem.: On the pathology of fragmentatio myocardii and myocarditis fibrosa. *Bull. Johns Hopkins Hosp., 9:*194-195, 1898.

Idem.: On the histogenesis of the striated muscle fibre and the growth of the human sartorius muscle. *Ibid., 9:*208-215, 1898.

Major, Ralph H.: *Classic Descriptions of Disease.* Springfield, Thomas, 1932. (pp. 630.)

Malloch, A.: *Short years.* Chicago, Normandie House, 1937.

Osler, W.: Harvey and his discovery. Harveian oration, Royal College of Physicians, London, 1906. In *An Alabama Student.* Oxford, Clarendon Press, 1909. (pp. 334)

Poiseuille, J. L. M.: Récherches sur la force du coeur aortique. Paris, Thèse. N. 166, 1828. (pp. 45.)

Poiseuille, J. L. M.: Récherches experimentales sur le mouvement des liquides dans les tubes de très petite diamètres. *C. R. Acad. Sci., 11:*961-967; 1041-1048, 1840. *Ibid., 12:*112-115, 1841. *Ibid., 16:*60, 1843.

Raynaud, M.: *On Local Asphyxia and Symmetrical Gangrene of the Extremities.* Translated by Thomas Barlow, M.D. London, New Sydenham Society, 1888. (pp. 150.)

Stirling, W.: *Some Apostles of Physiology.* London, Waterlow & Sons, 1902.

White, P. D.: In memoriam. Thomas Lewis. *Am. Heart J., 29:*419-420, 1945.

Willius, F. A., and Dry, T. J.: *A history of the heart and the circulation.* Philadelphia, W. B. Saunders, 1948. (pp. 456.)

Chemistry

Black, Joseph: *Treatise on Chemistry.* 1803, vol. II. (p. 87.)

Blake, J.: Mémoire sur les effets de diverse substances salines injectées dans le système circulatoire. *Arch. Gen. Med., 6:*289-300, 1839.

Cameron, H. C.: Patrick Playfair Laidlaw. *Guy's Hosp. Rep., 90:*1-14, 1940-41.

Cowgill, G. R.: Frederick Gowland Hopkins. *J. Nutrition, 40:*1-7, 1950.

Foster, M.: *Lectures on the History of Physiology.* Cambridge, University Press, 1924.

Giuseppi, J. A.: Families of long service at the Bank of England. *Genealogists' Mag., 10:*12, 1949.

Harris, H.: *California's Medical Story.* Springfield, Thomas, 1932. (421 pp.)

Hopkins and Biochemistry. 1861-1947. Cambridge, W. Heffer & Sons, 1949. (pp. 361)

Kendall, J.: *Great Discoveries by Young Chemists.* London, Nelson & Sons, 1953. (231 pp.)

Leake, C. D.: Gold Rush Doctor. *Gesnerus, 8:*114-123, 1951.

Marquardt, Martha: *Paul Ehrlich.* New York, Henry Schuman, 1951. (255 pp.)

Obituary Notice on Ehrlich. *The Times,* London, 20 August, 1915.

Osler, W.: *Biblioteca Osleriana.* London, Oxford University Press, 1929, p. 116. Notes on 1145, a copy of Black's thesis, which had belonged to James Syme and later to his son-in-law, Joseph Lister.

Ramsay, W.: *The Gases of the Atmosphere.* London, Macmillans, 1905.

Rhoads, C. P.: Paul Ehrlich and the cancer problem. *Ann. N.Y. Acad. Sci., 59:*190-197, 1954.

Sherrington, C. S., and others: Obituary notices of F. G. Hopkins. *Lancet, 1:*728-731, 1947.

Stirling, W.: *Some Apostles of Physiology.* London, Waterlow & Sons, 1902. (pp. 129)

Digestion

Babkin, B. P.: *Pavlov. A biography.* Chicago, University of Chicago Press, 1949. (365 pp.)

Bard, P.: Walter Bradford Cannon's Contributions to Physiology. In *W. B. Cannon—A memorial exercise.* Harvard Medical School, Nov. 5, 1945. (pp. 11-12.)

Bernard, C.: Du suc gastrique et de son rôle dans la nutrition. Paris, Thèse, 1843.

Bernard, C.: Récherches anatomiques et physiologiques sur la corde du tympan, pour servir à l'histoire de l'hemiplégie faciale. *Ann. Med.-psychol., 1:*408, 1843.

Cannon, W. B.: *Bodily Changes in Pain, Hunger, Fear and Rage.* New York, Appleton, 1915. (311 pp.)

Idem.: *The Wisdom of the Body.* New York, Norton, 1932. (327 pp.)

Idem.: *The Way of an Investigator.* New York, Norton, 1945. (229 pp.)

Catchpole, H. R.: Regnier de Graaf: Life and Works. *Bull. Hist. Med., 8:*1261-1300, 1940.

Foster, M.: *Claude Bernard.* London, T. Fisher Unwin, 1899. (245 pp.)

Foster, M.: *Lectures on the History of Physiology*. London, Cambridge, 1924. (306 pp.)

Frank, M.: History of the discovery of the secretory glands and their function. *Bull. Johns Hopkins Hosp., 27:*302-310, 1916.

Frolov, Y. P.: *Pavlov and his School.* London, Kegan Paul, 1937. (291 pp.)

Hemmeter, J. C.: Photography of the human stomach by the Roentgen method. *Boston Med. & Surg. J.*, June 18, 1896.

Hurst, Sir Arthur: *A Twentieth Century Physician.* London, Arnold, 1949. (200 pp.)

Kelly, Howard A.: John Richardson Young, Pioneer American Physiologist. *Bull. Johns Hopkins Hosp., 29:*186-191, 1918.

Meek, W. J.: Walter B. Cannon. An appreciation. *Texas Reports Biol. & Med., 11:*24-45, 1953.

Mendel, L. B.: An American contribution to the history of the physiology of digestion. *Popular Sc. Monthly, 74:*174-183, 1909.

Miller, W. S.: Niels Stensen. *Bull. Johns Hopkins Hosp., 25:*44-51, 1914.

Young, J. R.: An experimental enquiry into the principles of nutrition and the digestive process. M.D. thesis, University of Pennsylvania. In: *Medical Theses,* Ed. Charles Caldwell. Philadelphia, Thos. and Wm. Bradford, 1805.

Endocrines

Cave, A. J. E.: Richard Owen and the Parathyroid Glands. In: *Science, Medicine and History*. London, Oxford Univ. Press, 1953. (ii:217-222.)

Cohen, Sir Henry: Pierre Marie 1853-1940. *Proc. Roy. Soc. Med., 46:* 1047-1054, 1953.

Fraser, A. M.: Diuretic action of the oxytocic hormone of the pituitary gland. *J. Pharmacol., 60:*89, 1937.

Morrison, H.: Contributions to the microscopic anatomy of the pancreas by Paul Langerhans. *Bull. Inst. Hist. Med., 5:*259-265, 1937.

Seipel, C. M.: An English translation of Sandström's Glandulae Parathyreoideae. *Bull. Hist. Med., 6:*179-222, 1938.

Infection and Pathology

Camac, C. N. B.: *Epoch-making Contributions to Medicine, Surgery and the Allied Sciences.* Philadelphia, Saunders, 1909. (435 pp.)

Drewitt, F. Dawtrey: *Life of Edward Jenner.* London, Longmans Green, 1933. (151 pp.)

Edgar, I. I.: Ignaz Philipp Semmelweis. Outline for a biography. *Ann. Med. History, 1:*74-96, 1939.

Forbus, W. D.: William George MacCallum. 1874-1944. *J. Path. & Bact., 66:*603-607, 1944.

Hale-White, Sir Wm.: Translation of selected passages from De l'auscultation médiate, by R. T. H. Laennec with a biography. London, John Bale Sons, 1923. (193 pp.)

Kisch, B.: David Gruby. 1810-1898. *Trans. Amer. Phil. Soc., 44:*193-226, 1954.

Murphy, F. P.: Ignaz Philipp Semmelweis. An annotated bibliography. *Bull. Hist. Med., 20:*653-707, 1946.

Osler, W.: The Somerville Lectures. Natural History Society of Montreal. *Canad. J. Med. Sci. Toronto, 1:*134-135, 175-176, 1876.

Osler, W.: Influence of Louis on American Medicine. *Bull. Johns Hopkins Hosp., 8:*161-167, 1897.

Paget, Sir James: *Memoirs and letters.* London, Longmans Green, 1901. (pp. 55, 57.)

Rich, A. R.: William George MacCallum, 1874-1944. *Bull. Johns Hopkins Hosp., 75:*73 80, 1944.

Rouxeau, A.: *Laennec avant 1806.* Paris, Ballière, 1912. (295 pp.)

Thayer, W. S.: On some unpublished letters of Laennec. *Bull. Johns Hopkins Hosp., 31:*425-435, 1920.

Tilton, E. M.: *Amiable Autocrat; A biography.* (Oliver Wendell Holmes.) New York, Schumann, 1947.

Wiese, E. R.: Semmelweis. *Ann. Med. Hist., 2:*80-88, 1930.

Zakow, S. J.: Daniel A. Carrion of Carrion's Disease. *Quart. Bull. Northwest. Univ. Med. Sch., 17:*194-195, 1943.

The Lymphatics

Fulton, J. F.: The early history of the lymphatics. *Bull. Hennepin County Med. Soc., 9:*5-10, 1938.

Idem.: Charles Darwin (1758-1778) and the history of the early use of digitalis. *Bull. N.Y. Acad. Med., 10:*496-506, 1934.

Larsell, O.: Olof Rudbeck the Elder. *Ann. Med. Hist., 10:*301-313, 1928.

Nielsen, A. E.: A translation of Olof Rudbeck's Nova Excercitatio Anatomica. *Bull. Hist. Med., 11:*304-339, 1942.

Stirling, W.: *Some Apostles of Physiology.* London, Waterlow & Sons, 1902. (pp. 129.)

Von Hofstein, Nils: Olaus Rudbeck, in *Swedish men of Science,* edited by Sten Lindroth, Stockholm, The Swedish Institute, Almquist and Wiksell, 1952. (pp. 295.)

Nervous System

Alexander, Franz: Sigmund Freud, 1856-1939. *Arch. Neurol. & Psychiat., 43:*575-580, 1940.

Babkin, B.: *Pavlov. A Biography.* Chicago, Univ. Chicago Press, 1949. (365 pp.)

Berlin, R.: Beitrag Zur Strukturlehre der Grosshirnwindungen. Dis.-sert. Erlangen, A. E. Junge, 1858. (27 pp. 2 pl.)

Brain, W. R.: Presidential Address. Royal College of Physicians, London, Harrison & Son, 7 April 1952, p. 21.

Bravais, L. F.: Récherches sur les symptômes et le traitment de l'épilepsie hemiplegique. Thesis. Paris, Faculty of Medicine, 1827.

Claude, Henri: Les lesions du foie et les reins déterminées par certaines toxines. *Arch. de Physiol.* (Paris), *29:*843-847, 1897.

Dax, Marc: Lesions de la moitié gauche de l'encéphale coincidant avec l'oubli des signes de la parole. Thesis. Montpellier, 1836.

De Jong, R.: George Huntington. *Ann. Med. Hist., 9:*201-210, 1937.

Fulton, J. F.: *Selected Readings in the History of Physiology.* Springfield, Thomas, 1930. (p. vii.)

Idem.: A note on Francesco Gennari and the early history of cyto-architectural studies of the cerebral cortex. *Bull. Inst. Hist. Med., 5:*895-913, 1937.

Idem.: Sir Charles Scott Sherrington, O.M. *J. Neurophysiol., 15:*167-190, 1952.

Gennari, F.: De peculiari structura cerebri nonnullisque ejus morbis. Paucae aliae anatom. observat. accedunt, Parma, Regio Typographeo (Bodoni). 1782. (xvi. 87 p., 4 pl.)

Gibson, W. C.: Sherrington's Contribution to English Literature. *McGill Med. J., 17:*17-22, 1948.

Hassin, G. B.: Neuropathology—An historical sketch. *J. Neuropath. & Exper. Neurol., 9:*1-17, 1950.

Head, Henry: On the regulation of respiration. *J. Physiol.*, London, *10:*1-70, 279-290, 1889.

Jefferson, Sir Geoffrey: The Prodromes to cortical localization. *J. Neurol. Neurosurg. & Psychiat., 16:*59-72, 1953.

Jelliffe, S. E.: Sigmund Freud as a neurologist. *J. Nerv. & Ment. Dis., 85:*696-711, 1937.

John, H. J.: Jan Evangelista Purkyně, Czech scientist and patriot. *Proc. Roy. Soc. Med., 46:*933-940, 1953.

Jones, Ernest: *The life and work of Sigmund Freud.* New York, Basic Books, 1953. (428 pp.)

Kisch, Bruno: Forgotten leaders in modern medicine: Valentin, Gruby, Remak, Auerbach. *Trans. Amer. Philos. Soc. N.S., 44:*137-317, 1954.

Liddell, E. G. T.: Charles Scott Sherrington. Obituary Notices of Fellows of the Royal Society, *8:*241-270, 1952.

Marie, P.: Formes Frustes of Basedow's (Grave's) disease. Thesis. Paris, Faculty of Medicine, 1883.

Miles, A.: The Dynasty of the Monros. *Univ. Edinburgh J., 1:*54, 1925-6.

Olmsted, J. M. D.: *Charles Édouard Brown-Séquard.* Baltimore, Johns Hopkins Press, 1946. (253 pp.)

Overholser, W.: An historical sketch of psychiatry. *J. Clin. Psychopath., 10:*1-18, 1949.

Paget, Stephen: *Sir Victor Horsley. A Study of his Life and Work.* London, Constable, 1919. (358 pp.)

Russel, C. K.: Constantin von Monakow. 1853-1930. *Arch. Neurol. & Psychiat., 33:*1088-1097, 1935.

Strong, Nathan: *Inaugural Dissertation on the Disease Termed Petechial or Spotted Fever.* Hartford, Gleason, 1810.

Waller, A. V.: Microsopic examination of some of the principal tissues of the animal frame, as observed in the tongue of the living frog, toad, etc. *Philos. Mag., 29:*271-287, 397-405, 1846.

Idem.: Experiments on the section of the glosso-pharyngeal and hypoglossal nerves of the frog. *Phil. Trans. Roy. Soc. London,* 423-430, 1850.

Wiese, E. R.: Theodore Billroth, Scholar, Musician and Master Surgeon. *Ann. Med. Hist., 10:*278-286, 1928.

Young, A. W.: Franz Nissl and Alois Alzheimer. *Arch. Neurol. & Psychiat., 33:*847-852, 1935.

Physics and Optics

Bast, T. H.: *The Life and Times of Adolf Kussmaul.* New York, Hoeber, 1926. (137 pp.)

Chance, Burton: The early years of Helmholtz. *Am. J. Ophthalmol., 34:*1413-1420, 1951.

Darwin, F.: *Life and Letters of Charles Darwin.* London, vol. 3, 1887.

Fahie, J. J.: *Galileo, his Life and Works.* London, J. Murray, 1903. (451 pp.)

Forbes, H. S., and Wolff, H. G.: Cerebral Circulation. *Arch. Neurol. & Psychiat., 19:*1057-1086, 1928.

Govi, G.: The compound microscope invented by Galileo. *J. Roy. Microsc. Soc., 9*:574-598, 1889.

Lewis, Thomas: Obituary notice on Willem Einthoven. *Brit. Med. J., 2*:664-665, 1927.

McKendrick, J. G.: *Hermann Ludwig Ferdinand von Helmholtz.* London, Fisher Unwin, 1899. (299 pp.)

Oldham, Frank: *Thomas Young, F.R.S., Philosopher and Physician.* London, Edward Arnold, 1933. (159 pp.)

Sherrington, Sir Charles: *The Endeavour of Jean Fernel.* Cambridge, University Press, 1946. (223 pp.)

Watts, G. F.: Obituary notice on F. C. Donders. *Proc. Roy. Soc. London, 49*:7-24, 1891.

Index